N.N. Ergasheva
Jo.N. Majidova

Abnormal development of the spinal cord and spine in children

N.N. Ergasheva
Jo.N. Majidova

Abnormal development of the spinal cord and spine in children

ScienciaScripts

Imprint

Any brand names and product names mentioned in this book are subject to trademark, brand or patent protection and are trademarks or registered trademarks of their respective holders. The use of brand names, product names, common names, trade names, product descriptions etc. even without a particular marking in this work is in no way to be construed to mean that such names may be regarded as unrestricted in respect of trademark and brand protection legislation and could thus be used by anyone.

Cover image: www.ingimage.com

This book is a translation from the original published under ISBN 978-620-4-71796-8.

Publisher:
Sciencia Scripts
is a trademark of
Dodo Books Indian Ocean Ltd. and OmniScriptum S.R.L Publishing group
Str. Armeneasca 28/1, office 1, Chisinau-2012, Republic of Moldova, Europe
Printed at: see last page
ISBN: 978-620-5-27123-0

Contents

Foreword

The monograph considers measures on diagnostics, treatment and rehabilitation of patients with spinal dysraphism, on definition of separate kinds of myelodysplasia in structure of spinal and spinal cord anomalies; development of diagnostic criteria of disorders of pelvic organs function; estimation of significance of "fixed spinal cord" syndrome in genesis of residual disorders and dynamics of neurological disorders at stages of complex treatment; improvement of prevention of neurological displays of functional character and residual disorders and

The monograph is intended for neurologists and allied health practitioners, as well as undergraduate and postgraduate students.

INTRODUCTION

Relevance and relevance of the thesis topic. Spinal dysraphism occupies one of the leading places in the structure of spinal pathology of traumatic, infectious, tumor genesis and among malformations of the central nervous system (CNS). According to the World Health Organization, "spinal dysraphism in ethnic groups is 4.7 cases per 10,000 births. In the USA and a number of other countries it has not fallen below 3.4 cases per 10,000 live births, despite regular use of folic acid and other preventive measures. According to the State Statistics Service of the Russian Federation, diseases and anomalies in the development of the nervous system account for 21 - 18.5% of children with disabilities"[1].

The study of spinal dysraphism, its clinical and neurological aspects, and the optimisation of new approaches to diagnosis and improved treatment outcomes have been the subject of focused research worldwide. In particular, the early detection of hidden forms of spinal dysraphism using modern diagnostic methods makes it possible to improve surgical treatment tactics and reduce the risk of developing secondary spinal cord fixation syndrome. Identification of particular types of myelodysplasia within spinal and spinal cord anomalies in children; evaluation of the course and clinical manifestation of neurological and functional disorders associated with spinal dysraphism; identification of hidden forms and assessment of their role in the occurrence of neurological disorders in myelodysplasia and its combinations with urogenital and coloproctological anomalies; development of diagnostic criteria for pelvic organ function disorders are considered to be actual problems. It is recognized that the optimization of early comprehensive therapeutic system for vertebromedullary and combined anomalies with spinal cord lesions can reduce the risk of neurological deficits and improve the quality of life of patients.

---

1 World Health Report Geneva : World Health Organization. Available from URL:http://who.int/ whr /2014/en/statistics.htm;2014. Boulet SL, Yang Q, Mai C, Kirby RS, Collins JS, Robbins JM, et al. Trends in the postfortification prevalence of spina bifda and anencephaly in the United States. Birth Defects Res A Clin Mol Teratol 2008;82:527-32.

Uzbekistan's health care system is currently implementing a set of measures aimed at the early detection of anomalies of the nervous system in children and at reducing the incidence of complications. In this area, evidence-based results are needed to improve the system of medical care and the quality of diagnosis. **The action strategy for the five priority development areas of the Republic of Uzbekistan for 2017-2021 sets out the tasks** of developing and improving the system of medical and social care for children to ensure their full functioning[2] . Accordingly, the study of the clinical and paraclinical characteristics of spinal dysraphism in children and the optimization of medical care are relevant areas of scientific research. Adequate rehabilitation and social adaptation of patients in this group largely depends on timely diagnosis and comprehensive treatment of all existing disorders.

This dissertation work is aimed at solving the tasks stipulated by Presidential Decrees No. UP-4947 of 7 February 2017 "On the strategy for the further development of the Republic of Uzbekistan", No. PP-3071 of 20 June 2017 "On measures for the further development of specialized medical care for the population of Uzbekistan for 2017-2021", No. PP-2221 of 1 August 2014 "On the state programme for maternal, child and adolescent health in the Republic of Uzbekistan for 2014-2018" and other regulatory and legal documents

Compliance of the study with the priority directions of development of science and technology of the republic. Dissertation research was carried out in accordance with the priority direction of development of science and technology of the republic V1 "Medicine and Pharmacology".

Review of foreign scientific research on the topic of the thesis[3] **.**

Scientific research on the clinical and paraclinical characteristics of neurological disorders of the spinal cord in children, their diagnosis and treatment are carried

---

2 **Action Strategy for the Five Priority Development Areas of the Republic of Uzbekistan 2017-2021**

3   3 A review of international research on the topic of this thesis is based on https://www.aans.org/; https://www.chop.edu/centers-programs/center-fetal-diagnosis-and-treatment;https://www.university-directory.eu/   United-States-USA/   Childrens-Hospital-of-Philadelphia-and-the-University-of-Pennsylvanias-School-of-Medicine--Research-Institute.html;https://www.gradschools.com/programs/neuroscience; http://www.unifesp.br; https://www.nsi.ru/; http://www.almazovcentre.ru; http://neuro.uz and other websites.

out in leading medical centres and institutions of higher education in many countries around the world. These include the American Association of Neurological Surgeons (USA), Center for Fetal Diagnosis and Treatment, Children's Hospital of Philadelphia and the University of Pennsylvania School of Medicine, Philadelphia, Pennsylvania, (USA), Neural Development Unit, Institute of Child Health (London), Department of Paediatric Surgery, University Childrens Hospital Zurich, (Switzerland), Graduate Program in Neurology and Neurosurgery, Universidad Federal de São Paulo (UNIFESP), São Paulo, SP, Brazil (Brazil); Vanderbilt Institute of Neurosurgery, Universidad Federal de São Paulo (UNIFESP), São Paulo, SP (Brazil); Neurological Research Institute, São Paulo, SP. Acad. N. N. Burdenko Research Institute of Neurosurgery, Russian Academy of Medical Sciences (Russia), A.L. Polenov Research Institute of Neurosurgery (Russia), Specialized Research and Practice Medical Center of Neurosurgery, Ministry of Health of the Republic of Uzbekistan.

Promising results have been obtained in studies on the early diagnosis of cystic and occult forms of spinal pathology and the improvement of treatment tactics. These include: the introduction of antenatal ultrasound and MRI examinations made it possible to determine indications for surgical correction to prevent the aggravation of anatomical disorders and neurological consequences of the spinal cord after intervention in utero (Center for Fetal Diagnosis and Treatment, Children's Hospital of Philadelphia, (USA)); the high concurrence of spinal pathology in urinary tract and anorectal anomalies of polymorphic nature was revealed (Russian Research Institute of Neurosurgery named after prof. The influence of concomitant diseases on quality of life and death in children with spinal dysraphism has been demonstrated (Universidad Federal de São Paulo, Brazil); a direct relationship of neurological status and its dynamics with the nature and severity of spinal dysraphism has been revealed (Tashkent Pediatric Medical Institute).

At present in different countries scientific research on diagnostics, treatment and rehabilitation of patients with spinal dysraphism is being carried out in the following priority directions: determination of particular types of myelodysplasia in the structure of spinal and spinal cord anomalies; development of diagnostic criteria of pelvic organ dysfunction; assessment of significance of "fixed spinal cord" syndrome in genesis of residual disorders and dynamics of neurological disorders during complex treatment stages; perfection of neurolactic prevention.

Adequate rehabilitation and social adaptation of patients in this group largely depend on the timely diagnosis and comprehensive treatment of all disorders. However, neurological manifestations and residual functional impairments due to spinal insufficiency remain in many patients.

Extent of study of the problem. Numerous studies on early postnatal surgical correction and the development of modified surgeries for spinal cord and spine anomalies are ongoing (Chong Hyeok Yoon et al., 2014; Lora Kahn et al., 2014). Most works on the diagnosis and treatment of myelodysplasia reflect the surgical aspects of the treatment of spinal hernias or resulting urodynamic, colodynamic complications and locomotor disorders separately (Kolesnikova N.G.,2004; Khachatryan V.A. et al., 2009; Baindurashvili A.G. et al., 2013; Lazishvili M.N., 2014; Akhmediev M.M., 2013).

The introduction of antenatal ultrasound and MRI scanning has determined indications for surgical correction to prevent the aggravation of anatomical abnormalities and neurological consequences of the spinal cord after intervention in utero. Advances in this area include antenatal surgical correction of myelodysplasia using endovascular technology. Although the results do not always live up to expectations, researchers from various countries continue to look in this direction (Danzer E. et al., 2008; Scott Adzick N., 2010; Tereza Cristina Carbonari de Faria, Sergio Cavalheiro, 2013).

The lumbosacral spine accounts for 87% of the various forms of occult spinal dysraphism (OSD) in the form of spina bifida occulta (Voronov V.G. et al., 2016). Some authors consider this condition to be a variant of normal, as it is often asymptomatic and is a "finding" in the radiological examination of the spine.

Only subsequent anatomical studies and radiological data allowed the detection of concomitant changes in the sites of vertebral arches defect, which lead to nocturnal urinary incontinence, pain in the lumbosacral region, and posture disorders.

These changes have caused neurosurgeons and specialists to pay more attention to this pathology. A review of the literature shows a lack of attention to the detection of hidden forms of spinal dysraphism and the active treatment of neurological disorders and organ dysfunctions. According to current views, the complex treatment of congenital spinal pathology is aimed not only at providing a cosmetic effect and eliminating a specific anomaly, but also at correcting other associated anomalies, functional and organic disorders, and related complications (Martynenko A.A., Pislakov A.V. et al.) There are virtually no works on an integrated approach to diagnosis, treatment and rehabilitation of children with vertebromedullary anomalies.

Relationship of the thesis research with the plans of scientific and research work of the higher educational institution where the thesis was carried out. Dissertation research was carried out in accordance with the plan of research work of Tashkent Pediatric Medical Institute on the theme: "Improvement of diagnosis, treatment and prevention of congenital and acquired diseases in children" (2012-2016).

The aim of the study is to optimise early diagnosis, treatment and improve the quality of life of children with spinal cord and spinal cord abnormalities.

Research objectives:

To determine the nature and type of individual variants of myelodysplasia in the structure of spinal and spinal cord anomalies in children;

To identify the features of the course and clinical manifestation of neurological and functional disorders in children with spinal dysraphism;

Develop a diagnostic algorithm for spinal dysraphism in children;

To identify forms of occult spinal dysraphism and assess their role in the occurrence of neurological and functional disorders in myelodysplasia; their combination with urogenital and coloproctological abnormalities;

to assess the condition, types of impairment of the act of urination and colodynamics; to develop diagnostic criteria for pelvic organ dysfunction in vertebromedullary anomalies in children;

To assess the significance of fixed spinal cord syndrome in the genesis of residual impairment and the dynamics of neurological disorders during the stages of complex treatment;

Evaluate the effectiveness of early diagnosis and treatment measures involving specialist staff.

Subjects: 321 children with vertebromedullary anomalies of the spine and spinal cord, of whom 77 children were included in the retrospective study; a prospective study was conducted in 244 patients.

Subject: comprehensive assessment of the patient's somatic, neurological status and the anatomical and functional state of individual organs and systems using ultrasound, functional, radiological and special diagnostic methods.

Research methods. General clinical, laboratory, ultrasound, X-ray, computed tomography, magnetic resonance tomography, neurophysiological and statistical methods were used in the study.

The scientific novelty of the thesis research is as follows:

For the first time in the country, the frequency and nature of individual anomalies of the spine and spinal cord have been established;

The course, clinical manifestations and nature of organ disorders in overt and covert forms of myelodysplasia are systematised on the basis of comprehensive research data;

The neurological status and dynamics of spinal dysraphism before and during surgical treatment were studied; a direct correlation was found between the severity and polymorphism of the disorders and the nature and severity of the spinal dysraphism;

A frequent combination of occult spinal dysraphism and its role in the occurrence of neurofunctional abnormalities in anorectal, urogenital and coloproctal anomalies has been proven;

The genesis of residual and neurological disorders after operations for spinal malformations has been found to be dominated by the phenomenon of "fixed spinal cord syndrome" combined with congenital pathology or an adhesive process associated with the operation;

The need for a multidisciplinary approach to surgical and conservative treatment involving a paediatric neurologist, surgeon, urologist and orthopaedist has been demonstrated.

The practical results of the study are as follows:

Analysis of the incidence and types of spinal dysraphism proves the usefulness of comprehensive studies for their verification involving narrow specialists;

The diagnostic algorithm developed allows us to determine indications for staged examination by functional, ultrasound, radiation and special research methods to identify clinical, neurological, organ and functional disorders, which is necessary in practical health care;

the involvement of specialists in the comprehensive treatment and rehabilitation of children with vertebromedullary anomalies improves immediate and long-term outcomes;

persistent neurological symptoms against a background of conservative therapy is an indication for an MRI scan to detect "fixed spinal cord" syndrome and to determine the indication for reoperation;

A comprehensive examination during the stages of treatment enables the best rehabilitation programme to be devised, taking into account neurological and organ-functional disorders;

The results of the research are presented in the form of two methodological recommendations and have been introduced in the practice of paediatric neurological, surgical and orthopaedic departments of national and city medical institutions.

The validity of the results of the study is based on the application of theoretical approach and methods in the work, methodological correctness of conducting scientific research, sufficiency of the number of patients, conducting modern, complementary clinical and neurological, ultrasound, radiation and special research methods, study of new approaches to the diagnosis of spinal pathology, conclusion, the results were confirmed by the authoritative structures.

Scientific and practical significance of the research findings.

The scientific significance of the results of the study lies in the fact that the provisions, conclusions and suggestions of the co-author significantly add to the knowledge of diagnosis, clinical and neurological features, the complex treatment of osteonerval anomalies and myelodysplasia in children.

 The practical significance of the work is that the diagnostic algorithm developed allows us to determine indications for staged examination by functional, ultrasound, radiation and special research methods. A comprehensive approach to treatment after surgical intervention, early correction of neurological and concomitant disorders taking into account the author's suggestions contribute to improving the results of treatment in children and allow determining the prognosis of the disease.

Implementation of the results of the study. Based on the results of a scientific study of the clinical and paraclinical aspects of spinal dysraphism and new approaches to its diagnosis, the following were approved:

methodological recommendations: "Optimization of diagnosis of osteonerval anomalies of the spine and spinal cord in children" (opinion of the Ministry of Health of the Republic of Uzbekistan, No. 8H-r/149 of 12 October 2017). These methodological recommendations allowed the development of further stages of diagnostic investigations for osteonerval anomalies;

guidelines: "Diagnosis and treatment of pelvic organ dysfunctions in spinal malformations in children" (conclusion of the Ministry of Health of the Republic of

Uzbekistan, No. 8H-r/151 of October 12, 2017). The developed methodological recommendations allow to verify the types of pelvic organ dysfunctions in spinal malformations in children and to choose a complex treatment.

The proposed diagnostic tactic increases the vigilance of physicians of various specialties for early detection of primary or secondary changes in spinal pathology, the occurrence of functional and autonomic disorders in association with abnormalities of other organs and systems. Economic efficiency of research consists in reduction of multiplicity and duration of complex treatment. The results of the study are used in the paediatric neurology departments of the TashPMI clinic, the clinical bases of the department of hospital paediatric surgery, the routine surgery department, the 2nd children's clinical surgical hospital in Tashkent and the paediatric neurosurgery department of the scientific-practical neurosurgery centre of the MHRAz.

Approbation of the results of the work. The results of the research were discussed at 4 international and 5 national scientific-practical conferences.

Publication of research results. A total of 33 scientific papers, including 17 articles in journals recommended by the Higher Attestation Commission of the Republic of Uzbekistan, of which 15 were published in national and 2 in foreign journals, were published on the topic of the thesis.

Structure and volume of the thesis. The thesis consists of introduction, 6 chapters, conclusion, conclusions, practical recommendations, list of references; it is presented on 192 pages of computer typing.

Chapter I

Aspects of the diagnosis and treatment of spinal dysraphism in children (literature review)

§ 1.1. Structure, incidence of spinal pathology, clinical and morphological variants of spinal dysraphism

The close anatomical and functional relationship of the brain, the peripheral and autonomic nervous system, and the involvement of spinal cord structures in various pathological processes occurring in the patient's body result in a variety of spinal pathologies (SP) in children. Often, SP occurs in conjunction with changes in the spine and is referred to as osteoneural anomaly (ONA) or vertebrogenic myelopathies (VM). Various pathological conditions of the spine and spinal cord in children often have similar clinical manifestations and typical patterns of development. The ability to compensate, characteristic of childhood, often leads to underestimation of the severity of the condition and inadequate choice of diagnostic and therapeutic tactics. Despite the different etiology, the main manifestations of vertebrogenic myelopathies are similar: complete or partial loss of arbitrary movements and sensitivity below the lesion level, disorders of pelvic organ functions. Nosological forms in this group include spinal cord infections (SCI), tumours, traumatic lesions, and malformations characteristic of patients with persistent neurological deficits [61; 24 p.]. MSIs with motor impairments, including limb paralysis, account for 17-25% of acute neuroinfective disease and mainly occur in children under 5 years of age. Acute infectious myelopathies, encephalomyelo-polyradiculopathies of viral and bacterial etiology predominate in the structure of SCI. Poliomyelitis is now extremely rare as a result of mass vaccination of the population. ILIS is both viral (56.8%), mainly enteroviral (up to 90%), and bacterial (5.3%) in nature. Despite improvements in the diagnosis and treatment of IZSM, fatal outcomes are not uncommon; the incidence of residual effects is as high as 30%, and with lesions of anterior motoneurons, organic disorders remain lifelong in almost all relapsed patients [86; pp. 3-28].

Tumours of the spinal cord arising from the substance of the spinal cord are rare in childhood. CM tumours can be primary neoplasms originating in the spinal cord, metastatic neoplasms originating in the soft tissue and localised in the episubdural space. The ratio of spinal to brain tumours is approximately 1:6. Mostly school-age children are affected. Spinal cord tumours are divided into intramedullary tumours originating in the spinal cord and extramedullary tumours originating from structures surrounding the spinal cord (roots, vessels, membranes, epidural tissue). The neurological picture of spinal cord tumours consists of a progressively progressive syndrome of transverse spinal cord or cauda equina; mechanical blockage of the subarachnoid space and focal symptoms, whose features depend on the tumour location and its nature. Sensitivity disorder is one of the earliest symptoms of a CM tumour (61; p. 24).

Disease of the spinal cord due to traumatic injury is called traumatic CM disease. Until recently, spinal cord injuries in children were considered to be an infrequent injury, accounting for no more than 2-3% of other fracture localisations in children. In the last decade, the statistical rate of spinal injuries in children has increased from 2.5% to 8.0%. This is explained by the increased activity of children and the increasing number of severe injuries, including traffic injuries [102; p.26]. Several stages of traumatic SM can be distinguished. The acute period (up to 2-3 days) is characterized by symptoms of spinal shock: loss of movement, sensitivity, tendon and visceral reflexes; reduced muscle tone. In the early period (2-3 weeks) reflex excitability is restored with transition to hyperreflexia; symptoms of Babinski, pathological foot signs, clonic activity appear; muscle tone increases. In the intermediate stage (2-3 months), flexor or extensor muscle tone predominates. Spasticity (spastic plegia), muscle hypotrophy may result in pressure sores, joint contractures, reflex bladder. The late period (3 months to 1 year) is accompanied by a gradual, unidirectional (improvement or deterioration) change in the condition. The residual (more than 1 year) period of consequences and residual phenomena is characterized by a formed new level of neurological functions, the character of which changes little in the future [111; p.

185]. The population incidence of congenital malformations, according to the WHO Expert Committee, ranges from 2.7% to 16.3% in different countries with an average of 4-6% [40; pp. 58-61]. Congenital malformations are an important medical and social problem. The relevance of their study is due to their significant share in the structure of infant and perinatal mortality and childhood disability [75; p. 5-24].

Neural tube defects are among the leading human congenital anomalies. Most of these patients are considered incurable and die at an early age. Anomalies of the central nervous system (CNS) account for 30% of the anomalies. Isolated forms predominate in their structure. Often there are combined anomalies of the nervous system and neural tube as part of a symptom complex of multiple malformations. They have a severe course and are accompanied by complications and long-term or lifelong disability (23 and 23.4%) [167; pp. 1-12]. Among neural tube malformations, spinal hernia, anencephaly, and encephalocele account for 65%, 25%, and 10%. CNS abnormalities account for over 30% of all malformations found in children. According to L.S. Medina et al (1999), myelodysplasia occurs in 3% of newborns. Internationally, they are associated with 5 to 15% of referrals to paediatric neurology departments. [34; pp. 24, 176; pp. 1-5].

Neural tube defects represent an extensive polyetiological group of disorders of early and late ontogenesis (Huidi C., Dixian J., 1980; Romero R., Pilu J., Genty F. 1994). Malformations of the spinal cord account for 18.5% of the pathology of the nervous system and occur in 0.4-4.2 cases per 1000 newborns [33; pp. 53-61, 63; pp. 1-24, 89; pp. 122-125]. The true incidence of individual malformations of the spinal cord has not been established, due to the difficulties of diagnosis and the different approaches to their registration. To date, there is no unified treatment among researchers regarding the incidence of occult spinal dysraphism, which depends on the region of the world and ethnic groups. Spina bifida occulta, often localized in the L5 to S1 vertebrae, is found in 17% of the general population and in 30% of children aged 1 to 10 years [17; pp. 11, 26; pp.

147-148]. Analysis of the incidence of spinal herniation showed marked geographic variability. In Ireland the incidence is 3-4 cases, in the British Isles - 2-3.5, and in Eastern Europe and the USA - 0.1-0.6 cases per 1000 births. The rates in France, Italy and Spain are similar: 5 out of 1,000 have spina bifida [43; pp. 80, 63; pp. 2-24].

According to Mark S. Greenberg (2001) spina bifida occulta occurs in 20-30% of newborns in the US; 5-10% of these have congenital hydrocephalus; in 80% of cases this complication develops during the first 6 months of life. [34; c.24]. In the United States, the rate of Spina bifida has not fallen below 3.4 per 10 000 live births, despite the use of folic acid and other preventive measures of possible causative factors. All expectant mothers took 0.4 mg/day of folic acid a month before and throughout the first trimester of pregnancy to reduce the risk of having a baby with a spinal cord defect. Similar tactics have been used in other countries [136; pp. 527-532,139; pp. 223-227,166; pp. 49-57].

According to the literature, the prevalence of congenital malformations in Russia currently ranges from 3% to 7% [95; pp. 112-116]. The maximum incidence of gross structural abnormalities is 80-85% among spontaneously aborted fetuses. The incidence of congenital malformations of the nervous system in individual regions of the Russian Federation ranged from 0.1 to 0.9 per 1,000 births; the most severe malformation of the spinal cord, spinal hernias, ranged from 1:3,000 to 1:10,000 live births [34; pp. 24, 37; pp. 85-87].

In Uzbekistan, CNS malformations account for 54.9%. An analysis of the causes of stillbirth has shown that, in the presence of CHD in stillbirths, 78.2% are CNS malformations [11; pp. 112-116, 55; pp. 6-9]. According to A.T. Matchanova, 32 types of congenital malformations were the cause of early neonatal mortality in 17.1% of cases [66; p.24]. Malformations of the nervous system accounted for 10.5%. A study by A.Sh. Shodiev et al. on the population of congenital neurosurgical anomalies among children in Samarkand Province found that the incidence of hydrocephalus, craniostenosis, craniocerebral and spinal hernias was 2 cases per 1000 births, more frequent among the urban population. According to their data, 18.5% of children with malformations of the nervous system were hospitalized at 4-7 months of age; 42% from 7 months to one year; 23.3% from one to three years. [113; c. 355].

Spinal dysraphism is a collective term that combines pathologies with a common mechanism of development, varied in the form of incomplete congestion of medially located mesenchymal, bone and nerve structures; often with latent clinical and neurological abnormalities of musculoskeletal, pelvic and other system functions. Osteonerval dysplasia occurs in any part of the spine. In compression of the dural sac through a bone defect, fixation of spinal roots or spinal cord sections, pronounced neurological symptoms are observed [5; pp. 10-13, 37; pp. 85-87].

Depending on the nature of the spinal cord disruption and the damage to the mesenchymal tissue in the area of the defect, several types of malformation are distinguished. Spinal dysraphism is manifested by an open cleavage of the spine with the formation of a cystic spinal hernia (spina bifida cystica uverta) (spina bifida aperta); a closed form (spina bifida occulta); cleavage of the spine and soft tissue with spinal cord splitting throughout or in a particular segment (rhachischiasis totalis et partialis) [64; pp. 133-137, 87; pp. 208-209, 156; pp. 13-22]. Among the open forms, the spinal hernia (SMH) deserves special attention. The most common form of SMH is cystic cleft of the spine (spina bifida cystica), a protrusion of the membranes, spinal nerve roots, and spinal cord in the area of spinal incomplete closure of the spinal canal. SMH is often combined with other malformations, particularly of the brain. It is more commonly located in the lumbosacral region and can range in size from small (the size of a walnut) to huge. If the bulge increases in size, the skin above it becomes thin and infected. The hernial bulge may rupture and spread infection through the liquor ducts of the spinal cord and brain. Depending on the contents of the hernial sac, the following forms of SMH can be distinguished. *A meningocele* is a protrusion of only the membranes of the spinal cord, filled with cerebrospinal fluid. A meningoradiculocele is characterised by the prolapse of thin, insufficiently myelinated spinal nerve roots, usually fused to the wall of the herniated sac, into the herniated sac. *Myelomeningocele: the* spinal cord bulges out along with the membranes and altered spinal nerve roots; *myelocystocele:* the central canal of the spinal cord is dilated and filled with cerebrospinal fluid; the spinal cord along with the membranes bulges out through a congenital defect in the spinal column [30; pp. 395, 43; pp. 80, 50; p. 304].

Spina bifida complicata is a combined neural tube formation pathology including various forms of spinal hernias and dystopic lipoma formation, fibrous tissue or with teratoid inclusions of heterogeneous structure around the herniated protrusion in cystic cleft. It is located under the skin, forms a defect in the vertebral arch, and may protrude into the meninges and fuse with the spinal nerve roots and spinal cord. The clinical picture of SMH consists of local changes and neurological disorders. The leading clinical syndromes in SMH are motor, pelvic, sensory, trophic and vegetovascular disorders [101; pp. 52-57, 106; pp. 15-23, 150; pp. 1-4, 200; pp. 476-483].

The lumbosacral spine accounts for 87% of the varied forms of occult spinal dysraphism (OSD) presented as spina bifida occulta. The only thing they have in common is the lack of skin integrity over the vertebral defect. In children, spina bifida occulta is varied in terms of both the number of cleft vertebrae and the associated spinal cord abnormalities with different clinical features. Initial symptoms often appear delayed and progress slowly; an MRI scan of the spinal cord is necessary to make a definitive diagnosis. [5; c. 26].

Signs of spinal cord damage are largely evident in adolescence or young adulthood. An external manifestation of occult forms may be the presence of hypertrichosis, angiomas, lipomas and skin traps in the defect area, which sometimes present as congenital sinuses: dermal or pilonidal. Congenital dysraphic malformations of the caudal spine and spinal cord can manifest as flaccid paralysis and paresis of the lower limbs; various sensory disorders; urinary and faecal incontinence; pronounced trophic changes, orthopaedic deformities, internal organ disorders. Symptoms may be absent for a long time and then suddenly develop after an injury, flu, or other provocation at any age. These disorders often lead to permanent disability of children and their social and labour disadaptation [54; p.47].

Some authors regard this condition as normal, because it is often asymptomatic and is an incidental "finding" in the radiological examination of the spine (29; p. 53-61). Some publications have previously stated that incomplete closure of the sacral arches occurs in 70% of people and is a normal phenomenon, characteristic of the phylogenesis of the human sacrum and the processes of its reduction and transverse extension during the transition from horizontal to vertical position (Speransky, 1925). According to Voronov (2002), this thesis of an authoritative scientist significantly decreased the physicians' attitude to spina bifida occulta as a manifestation of a congenital anomaly of the spinal cord and spine, which often required surgical treatment. Subsequent anatomical studies and radiological findings revealed concomitant changes at the sites of vertebral arches defect, leading to nocturnal urinary incontinence, pain in the lumbosacral region, posture disorders; less frequently, weakness of leg muscles, foot deformity, sensory and trophic disorders. The revealed changes convinced neurosurgeons in the necessity of surgical treatment at the onset of signs of pathology [64, p. 133-137, 98; p.197]. There may be no obvious symptoms with this abnormality. Some patients show symptoms of prolapse, irritation of the nervous system in the form of lumbosacral pain, hyperaesthesia, and paresthesias in the lower extremities. With a typical localization of spinal dysraphism in the lumbosacral region, a variety of vertebral anomalies combined with anorectal, urogenital, and colorectal abnormalities or dysfunction of these organs occur [56; p.24]. According to Kolesnikova N.G. (2005), spina bifida of the lumbosacral spine are combined with anorectal dysfunction in all cases. The author identifies physiological spina bifida posterior of the lumbosacral spine as a marker of morphofunctional immaturity of the neuromuscular apparatus of the anorectal zone, manifested by impaired vegetative innervation. Dysplastic spina bifida posterior is a marker of mixed (autonomic and somatic) neurological deficits in the anorectal zone. A variant of spina bifida is the anterior spinal hernia (spina bifida anterior), which is extremely rare and represents a developmental defect of the vertebral bodies.

Osteovertebral spinal anomalies may present as stenosis with a decrease in the anteroposterior dimension of the spinal canal in the lumbar region. Spinal canal stenosis is one of the most common congenital anomalies of the lumbar spine. It results from shortening and thickening of the lumbar vertebral arches. Reduced size of the canal may result in local compression of the nerve structures. The combination of spinal canal stenosis and prolapsed intervertebral disc leads to compression-ischemic lesion of the cauda equina and cone-epicondylar spinal cord (Vasilieva O.V., 2002; Ragimov O.Z., 1993). As a complication of chronic neural insufficiency of the lumbosacral plexus, prolapse and then prolapse of the vaginal and uterine walls in women develops [107; p. 304].

SSD **is a** heterogeneous group of malformations of the spine and spinal cord. The incidence of SSD is 0.05-0.25 cases per 1000 newborns and most cases are localised to the lumbosacral spine. The true incidence of SSD is unknown because its manifestations are not as pronounced as those of spinal hernias. (98; p. 28,161; p.71-79).

There are many publications on the diagnosis of caudal neural tube malformations. MRI, CT, ultrasound, and neurophysiological diagnostic methods are important in the examination of patients with manifestations of spinal dysraphism, in which various variants of spinal malformations related to occult spinal dysraphism are identified [14; pp. 413-415, 22; pp. 18, 57; pp. 175-178]. These include diastematomyelia (division of the spinal cord in length into two parts by a bone, cartilage, or fibrous bridge); diplomyelia (doubling of the spinal cord in the cervical or lumbar thickening; more rarely, the entire spinal cord doubles; both brains lie in the same bed consisting of soft and hard dura mater, in places connected by glial tissue, well developed and with all components of the spinal cord) hydromyelia (hydrocele of the spinal cord in which the spinal canal is dilated, lined with ependyma and filled with cerebrospinal fluid, usually thinning the spinal cord in the posterior columns); syringomyelia (with the formation of cystic cavities in the spinal cord as a communicating and non-communicating form). The incidence of syringomyelia varies from 0.3 to 8.4 per 100,000 population in different countries. The disease may be congenital or acquired as a result of spinal cord injury, tuberculous lesions, or a complication of spinal pathology. The congenital form of the disease is often familial and affects predominantly males (70; pp. 26, 72; pp. 245, 96; pp. 339-340). Amyelia, the complete absence of the spinal cord with preservation of the dura mater and spinal ganglia, has also been observed. On the place of spinal cord, sometimes there is a thin fibrous band [91; p. 119-120].

Spinal lipomas (SL), the most common form of occult spinal dysraphism, are subdivided into three groups: intradural, spinal cord cone lipomas; end-thread lipomas. Lipomas in the region of the spinal cord cone are in turn subdivided into: lipomyelocele - lipomatous tissue spreading from the substance of the spinal cord transdurally into the subcutaneous fatty tissue of the lumbosacral region; lipomyelomeningocele - subcutaneous meningomyelocele combined with lipoma; lipomyelocystocele - the terminal parts of the spinal cord are turned outward by cystic dilatation of the central canal [29; pp. 53-61, 43; c.80, 78; pp. 14-17, 178; pp. 84-87]. SLs in the cone or terminal filament region of the spinal cord are the cause of fixed spinal cord syndrome (SFSM). Cases of spinal lipomas unrelated to spinal dysraphism have been reported in the literature. They are more often localised in the thoracic region or involve extended areas of the spinal cord; they occur predominantly in adults. Among caudal malformations of the spinal cord, lipomeningocele accounts for 8-25% of cases [200; pp. 476-483, 202; pp. 1731-1739]. [169]. According to L Marca et al. 1997, lipomatous spinal masses account for 35% of lumbosacral masses; 20% of them are lipomeningocele. According to Voronov V.G., among 132 different forms of malformations of the spinal cord and spine, lipomas were observed in 11.5% of cases and accounted for less than 1% of spinal tumours. Spinal lipomas occur at a rate of 4-8 per 100,000 in the general population, more commonly in girls. Often the clinical presentation depends on the age and developmental period of the child. The average age of patients at diagnosis is 3-4 years [29; pp. 53-61]. Clinical manifestations of lipomeningocele in neonates are minimal. Approximately half of patients have their first symptoms after 6 months of life. As the child grows, neurological symptoms appear and gradually progress. Almost 90% of patients at the age of two years have neurological deficits. The low intensity of clinical manifestations in young children can be explained by the soft-elastic consistency of the tumor and its median and sparsely infiltrative growth [109; pp. 76-87, 110; p. 356]. The clinical manifestations of SL range from subtle signs to severe involvement of the spinal cord. The most common manifestations are urinary incontinence, foot deformities, asymmetric hypotrophy of the lower extremities with mosaic sensory disturbances. Back or lower limb pain is less common. In the diagnosis of spinal lipomas, MRI examinations have a sensitivity and specificity of 73.3% and 100%, while MSCT has a sensitivity of 68.4% and 100% [5; p. 22, 34; p. 24].

Chiari malformation (MC) is a chronic compression and displacement of cerebellar and brainstem structures into the greater occipital foramen and below, with impaired blood flow in the vertebrobasilar basin and liquor circulation in the craniovertebral area. The main pathomorphological substrate is herniation of the posterior and medulla oblongata extending into the cervico-occipital foramen and combined with herniation of any spinal region. The spinal cord fixed in the meningocele causes traction of the brain stem and cerebellum down into the cervo-occipital funnel with spinal growth. The development of hydrocephalus is secondary in this case. In about 80% of patients, MC is combined with spinal cord pathology and leads to complex craniospinal syndromes in the form of progressive myelopathy. The incidence ranges from 3.3 to 8.2 cases per 100,000 population [30; pp 395, 67; pp 49-52, 82; pp 331, 154; pp 1749-1752]. There are currently four types of MC, based on neuroimaging parameters. Type I is a congenital deformity of the hindbrain with prolapse of the cerebellar amygdala in the normal position of the IV ventricle, sometimes combined with a reduction in size or deformity. Type II is characterised by a congenital pathology of the hindbrain, which is almost always combined with a meningocele or meningomyelocele. Ectopia of the cerebellar vermis, ventricle IV and brain stem occur in this pathology; in more severe cases other cerebral anomalies and spinal dysraphism may also accompany it.

Type III and type IV anomalies are rare and are characterised by marked clinical manifestations. Cerebellar herniation with cervical encephalocele is identified in type III MC. Type IV MC is characterised by severe cerebellar agenesis and/or hypoplasia of the pons and spinal cord. Types I and II are more common. The pathology occurs in children of all age groups. The nature and severity of clinical and neurological disorders of blood and cerebrospinal circulation in the form of vegetovascular, hypertension-hydrocephalic, cerebellar, pyramidal, bulbar and spinal syndromes depend on the shift of the brain structures along the spinal canal in the caudal direction, the degree of spinal cord fixation and the nature of concomitant spinal pathology. Neurosonography, MSCT, and MRI examinations of the brain and spinal cord are used in diagnosis [175; pp. 20-35, 206; p. 8239]. The most informative method of diagnosis is MRI of the brain and spinal cord with determination of the relationship between bony and cerebral structures at the level of the craniovertebral junction. Neurophysiological studies allow us to assess the dynamics and nature of brain damage at the stages of treatment [201; pp. 311-316].

Many malformations of the caudal spine and spinal cord are complicated by fixed spinal cord syndrome (SFSM). In normal intrauterine development of the fetus in the third month the spinal cord occupies the entire length of the spinal canal. In the following months, the spinal cord grows faster than the spinal cord. As a result, in the newborn, the spinal cord ends at the level of the third lumbar vertebra and by the age of 12-18 months it only reaches the lower edge of the LI or upper edge of the LII vertebra. The term 'tethered spinal cord' (TSM) was coined by H.J. Hoffmann et al (1976). FSM can develop due to scarring and adhesions at the site of surgical interventions performed during the neonatal period. It concerns, first of all, congenital spinal hernia of lumbosacral localization [90; pp. 348-353, 91; pp. 119-120, 99; pp. 53-58]. In cases where the cone and epicondyle of the spinal cord are located below this level and the corresponding clinical symptomatology, the pathological component is considered as the tethered cord syndrome (TCS). The term is suggested by S. Yamada et al (1981). The authors found that tension and limitation of mobility of the spinal cord caused by its fixation in the lumbosacral spine lead to impaired metabolism and physiological activity of caudal neuronal formations [5; p.22]. It was proved that the pathophysiological basis of SFSM is the mechanical traction of the caudal spinal cord, accompanied by a decrease in blood flow in the involved area, resulting in ischemia, depression of electrical activity of the spinal cord, and, on the biochemical level, inhibition of oxidative phosphorylation in neuronal mitochondria [101; pp. 52-57]. In SFSM, pathological attachment of the spinal cord cone in the spinal canal limits its physiological mobility during flexion movements of the spine. As the child grows, this prevents age-related upward displacement of the spinal cord cone, which aggravates the disembryogenic manifestations of the existing neurological deficit. The signs of spinal cord "fixation" are a progressive increase in the existing or formerly absent dysfunctions of pelvic organs, sensory, motor, and trophic symptoms in the perineum and lower extremities [90; pp. 348-353, 109; 76-87, 133; pp. 13-17,151; pp. 93-97]. Magnetic resonance imaging is the leading method in the diagnosis of morphological signs of the syndrome. Echospondylography is indicated as a screening technique and is informative in detecting an abnormally low spinal cord cone.

Thus, SPSM brings together a group of diseases of congenital or acquired origin with common pathogenetic mechanisms caused by organ tension due to fixation of its caudal region due to an imbalance in the osteoneural development of the spinal cord and spinal column. Clinically, they are manifested by various combinations and intensities of motor, sensory, trophic, pelvic disorders; bone and joint deformities of the lower extremities; autonomic disorders and internal organ dysfunctions. From the current perspective, the spectrum of patients with SPSM includes children with spinal dysraphia, acquired post-traumatic, post-infection and other conditions in which there is fixation and tension of the caudal spinal cord. The group of congenital causes includes spinal dysraphisms, the common feature of which is intrauterine fixation of the spinal cord. The most common congenital causes are lumbosacral lipomas: lipomyelomeningocele, terminal filament lipomas and terminal medullary cone lipomas, dermal sinus tracts, diastomatomyelia, dorsal fixation bands in meningocele [47; pp 325-326, 91; pp 119-120, 97; pp 28, 98; pp 197, 203; pp 3850]. In acquired conditions, the source of fixation is scar tissue within the dural sac, most commonly occurring after surgical correction of spinal dysraphia. This condition is referred to as Secondary Spinal Cord Fixation Syndrome (SCSSS). One in three children after correction of a myelomeningocele needs 'spinal cord release' surgery due to the development of SPSSM. SPSM is observed not only in children, but also in adults [29; pp. 53-61, 59; 41-46, 149. p. 1503]. There are currently no reliable data on the incidence of this syndrome in a large population. In a single study, the incidence of SPSM was 0.1% in a series of 5,500 school-age children [107; pp. 304, 151; pp. 93-97].

Although there are descriptions of the clinical and morphological features of SFSM in the literature, certain aspects of this issue have not been resolved. In particular, the clinical presentation of fixed spinal cord syndrome, depending on its etiology, has not been sufficiently studied. The value of examination methods for patients with "fixed spinal cord" syndrome and the possibility of using them for screening newborns and older children have not been clarified. The indications for differentiated surgical treatment for spinal cord fixation in the spinal canal require clarification. The prevention of SPSM developing in response to surgical interventions in the caudal spine and spinal cord is insufficiently studied.

§ 1.2 Etio-pathogenetic aspects of spinal malformations

CNS malformations represent a large polyetiological group of disorders of early and late ontogenesis. They are caused by abnormalities in one or more basic processes of brain development: formation of the neural tube, division of its cranial part into paired formations; migration and differentiation of nerve cell elements. They manifest themselves at three levels: cellular, tissue and organ. This provision is fully applicable to the terminal brain and to a lesser extent to the stem sections, whose structural abnormalities may be the result of damage to the terminal brain. In most cases, their multifactorial nature can be established. Most authors consider disturbance of embryogenesis processes at the stage of neural and bone system formation from 16 days to the end of 8 weeks after fertilization, when not only the spine, but also the major internal organs are formed, to be possible etiological factors [40; pp.58-61]. Closing of the neural tube is usually completed within four weeks after conception, before the woman realizes she is pregnant. Anencephaly and spina bifida have been found to be overt defects of the neural tube, resulting from abnormalities in the formation of the primitive neural tube (63; pp. 24, 137; pp. 225-231).

External factors contributing to neural tube defects include: radiation, toxic chemicals (oil products, fertilizers, pesticides); use of anticonvulsants by a woman before pregnancy and in the first months; high body temperature or use of hot baths in early pregnancy; diabetes mellitus and obesity, unbalanced diet, vitamin deficiency, especially folic acid deficiency [10]. If there have been cases of children born with neural tube defects among close relatives, the chance of having a child with such a defect increases to 2-5%.

Bokonbaeva S.D. et al. (2010), based on the results of genealogical studies, found: hereditary forms of CMH in 18.8%, and a hereditary and family history in 100% of cases. Aggravating trigger risk factors in the formation of hereditary forms of neural tube malformations were identified, and the possibility of repeated birth of children with spinal hernia was noted. The clinical and genealogical analysis of neural tube pathology showed a burden of congenital and hereditary pathology in 9.7% of families. Malformations, including those of the nervous system, were found in 4.7% of the parents. The chromosomal and monogenic pathology was registered in the anamnesis in 0.8% and 0.3% of the families [40; pp. 58-61, 58; p.24, 99; pp. 53-58].

The initial state of health of the parents is important in the occurrence of congenital malformations in children. According to Voronov V.G., Syrchin E.F., Zyabrov A.A., unfavourable factors acting on the mother and foetus during pregnancy accounted for 65.2% of all factors studied. In 69.4% of mothers the course of pregnancy and childbirth was accompanied by various acute diseases (acute respiratory viral infections, influenza, sore throat, nasopharyngitis, bronchitis, acute gastritis, enteritis); it was more often complicated by urogenital tract infection and obstetric pathology. A higher incidence of threatened termination of pregnancy and prolonged gestosis throughout the pregnancy was noted [40; pp.58-61, 47; pp. 325-326]. A poor obstetric history was found in 46% of mothers, and a pathological course of pregnancy in 95%. Half of the women were found to have gynaecological disorders. Extragenital maternal pathology accounted for a significant proportion of premorbid risk factors (80%), with gastrointestinal diseases (25%), diseases of the visual organs (23%), endocrine and urinary systems predominating. Somatic diseases have various combinations in most cases (22 per cent).

Of equal importance among risk factors are urogenital infections, including those included in the TORCH complex, which were detected in 74% of women. Among the causative agents, ureaplasmosis accounted for 13.5%, herpes infection for 15%, and cytomegalovirus infection for 11%. The impact of biological and physicochemical factors on the fetus during the teratogenic terminal period has not been sufficiently studied. However, it has been shown that toxicosis and viral infectious diseases in women in the first half of pregnancy initiate the development of caudal myelodysplasia syndrome in 25% of cases [75; pp. 5-24, 126; pp. 9-14, 136; 527-532, 17, 19].

§ 1.3. Aspects of comprehensive diagnosis of spinal malformations

Congenital dysraphisms of the caudal spine and spinal cord in children can manifest as motor disorders in the form of flaccid paralysis and paresis of the lower extremities; disorders of sensory and pelvic organ function, the appearance of orthopedic deformities; trophic changes in various parts of the body and lower extremities [11; 112-116, 19; 97-102, 42; p. 324]. They are extremely diverse and polymorphic in children of all age groups. Most of them with obvious external manifestations are detected in the period of newborn and infant age. Some forms have latent or moderately pronounced neurological disorders and are detected in older children and adults by special research methods [150; pp. 1-4, 200; pp. 476-483]. Early diagnosis of SSD depends primarily on paediatricians' alertness to this pathology. The symptomatology of SSD is usually associated with fixed spinal cord syndrome, progressing as the child grows. More than 90% of patients have cutaneous stigmata of SSD: subcutaneous lipomas, angiomas, localised hairiness, dermal sinus. The use of clinical, electrophysiological, radiological, ultrasonographic methods and spinal MRI examinations make it possible to estimate the level of the spinal cord lesion and the type of anomaly [119; 322-323, 189; p. 2121]. Despite different etiologies, the main manifestations of vertebrogenic myelopathies are similar: complete or partial loss of arbitrary movements and sensitivity below the lesion level and disorders of pelvic organ function. Depending on the area of the SM lesion along the transverse plane, different symptoms are observed. Lesions in the anterior SM are accompanied by a loss of voluntary movements, pain and temperature sensitivity, but proprioceptive sensitivity is retained. Posterior SM lesions are characterised by loss of proprioceptive sensitivity, whereas voluntary movement, pain and temperature sensitivity are not affected. Complete transverse lesion of the SM is characterised by a lack of voluntary movements and all types of sensitivity. Half-small lesions are characterised by a loss of movement, vibration and proprioceptive sensation and touch on the affected side of the body and a conductive absence of pain and temperature sensation on the opposite side (Braun-Sekar syndrome). Neurological symptoms occur below the level of the lesion. An exception is ascending myelopathies, the pathogenesis of which is not associated with mechanical damage to the nervous structures, but with tractional myeloischemia. Microcirculatory changes in the spinal cord are located above the zone of spinal damage, which is clinically manifested by an inconsistency in the level of bone and neurological disorders. According to the number of limbs losing voluntary control of movements, mono-, para-, tri-, and tetraplegia can be distinguished; by severity, full or partial plegia can be distinguished [33; p.123-125]. Motor disturbances and loss of sensation are common neurological symptoms. A comparative analysis of the development of the lower extremities in normalborn and children with spinal cord and spinal cord abnormalities shows shortening of the length and circumference of the lower extremities, which can be considered a manifestation of trophic disorders as hypotrophy or atrophy of one or both extremities. These changes persist in both non-surgical and surgical patients [19; pp.27-29, 31; pp.17-22]. In the natural course of the disease or after surgery for a spinal hernia, various complications occur in some patients. Trophic ulcers and urogenital sepsis are a formidable consequence. Their pathogenesis is dominated by neurogenic disorders, accompanied by a sharp decrease in blood flow in the microvasculature of the affected part of the body, leading to ischaemia, hypoxia and tissue necrosis. There are very few publications on this subject [33; pp.123-125, 44; pp. 85-89,].

Pelvic disorders in the form of urinary and defecation disorders are considered to be important components of the clinical manifestations of osteonerval anomalies of the spine and spinal cord; they often determine the patient's degree of adjustment, the severity and prognosis of the disease. Dysfunction results from abnormalities in the suprasegmental and segmental nervous apparatus of the spinal cord. Anatomical and physiological peculiarities of the rectum, bladder and lower urinary tract, their close interconnection, and common innervation cause the development of combined disorders of pelvic organ function of organic and functional nature [42; p. 324, 84; pp. 47-51]. Instability in the act of urination or defecation can be due to the morpho-functional immaturity of the neuromuscular apparatus in young children. However, there is no doubt about the importance of osteoneural anomalies of the spine and spinal cord in the occurrence of anomalies, the progression of functional phenomena from the urinary tract and the anorectal zone, due to the commonality of their pathogenetic mechanisms (Bao Quan Qi, 2004; A. Holschneider, J. Hutson, 2006; A.D. Cesare 2010). The frequency of pelvic organ dysfunction, according to the literature, ranges from 68%, which cover only disorders of urination or the act of defecation without a detailed analysis of the combined disorders [82; p.28, 107; p.304]. Given synchronism, unity and interrelation of functions, it is impossible to consider separately pathophysiological processes in urogenital and coloproctologic systems. The results of complex treatment are not always comforting. Because of the failure of surgery and drug therapy, most children require repeated corrective surgeries.

The development of effective methods of correction of pelvic organ disorders in general and urological complications in particular is an urgent task for specialists in various medical disciplines (Komissarov I.A., 1996; Prityko A.G. et al., 1997; Voronov V.G., 2000; Kushel Y.A., 2003; Polunin V.S. et al. 2006; Guseva N.B. 2007; Michelson D.J., Ashwal S., 2004, Osipov I.B., Elikbaev G.M., 2009 Ergashev N.Sh., 2016). Only sporadic works of pediatric surgeons devoted to megacolon has considered the issue of combined pathology of spinal cord as a cause of developmental anomalies and chronic colostasis [41; pp.263-264, 59; pp.41-46, 122; pp.57-58]. .

According to some authors, 30-50% of children with spinal hernia sequelae develop subluxation or dislocation of the hip joint during the first 2-3 years of life. The type and severity of the detected abnormalities with deterioration or improvement with age depend on the level and extent of the neurosegmental lesion (Ivanov S.V., Kenis V.M., 2013; Erol B, et al., 2005; Baindurashvili A.G. et al. 2013). The mismatch between the growth of the sheaths and the spinal cord and the growing spine causes stretching of the nerve fibres, pressing against the strained dura mater. The result is impaired muscular balance, paresis or paralysis of the muscles of the lower extremities; decreased neutralisation of deforming forces in limb loads;

and deformed joints in the affected area of the spinal cord. These abnormalities may be congenital or appear in a child in later years with a progressive course [19; pp.97-102, 31; pp.17-22, 151; pp.93-97]. Disproportionate muscle traction, trophic effects, aggravating statico-dynamic factors without orthopaedic prevention aggravate deformities of the musculoskeletal system. Motor disorders (from complete loss of function or weakness of some muscle groups to increased tone of other muscle groups) cause various degrees of fixation and severity of individual components of the deformity. With a mild non-fixed deformity, passive elimination of its elements is possible; with a rigid one, surgical correction is necessary [172; pp. 350-353, 177; pp. 602-605]. Modern diagnosis of spinal pathologies in children involves a complex of clinical, instrumental, radiological and special methods of investigation, including computer and magnetic resonance imaging [12; pp. 55-56, 25; pp. 201-202, 34; pp. 24, 132; pp. 1832, 203; p. 3850]. The different informative value of instrumental methods of investigation for different spinal cord pathology requires the use of adequate methods or their sequence in each particular case. (Olin A.V., Makarov A.Yu., Mgurkevich E.A. 1995; Malchenko O.V., Danilevskaya I.M., Mushkin A.Yu. 2011) [42; c.324].

Prenatal diagnosis of malformations is currently gaining importance, with screening ultrasound being the main method. A review of the literature shows that a spinal hernia can be detected in the first trimester of pregnancy. The minimum time for diagnosis of this abnormality is noted in a study by Gao F. [3; pp. 73-76], who presented 3 cases of established diagnosis at 9-10 weeks. Other foreign specialists were able to do so at 12-14 weeks of gestation. Despite the widespread use of ultrasound, prenatal diagnosis of certain forms of spinal malformations remains difficult. According to foreign studies, their detection rate, on average, is no more than 45% [72; pp. 301-304]. The results of screening ultrasound examinations in various centres show that spina bifida is one of the most difficult to diagnose malformations [20; pp. 45-47].

In recent decades, antenatal screening of the fetus in the second and third trimesters of pregnancy has been performed. This makes it possible to determine the risk group for the development of irreversible changes, the tactics of pregnancy management, and the plan of treatment measures in the early postnatal period (Pislakov A.V. et al., 2008; José Murillo B. Netto, Maryland) [82;p 28, 161; pp.71-79]. Advances in antenatal diagnosis of spinal malformations using fetal ultrasound and fetal MRI have opened the possibility of corrective surgery endoscopically in myelodysplasia to prevent the progression of anatomical and neurological disorders in the fetus in utero. Tulipan and Bruner in 1997, Adzick and N.S. et al. in 1998 proved the feasibility of intrauterine open surgery at 28-30 weeks' gestation [126; pp. 9-14, 198; pp.27-33].

The main significance in the postnatal diagnosis of SM disease is the neurological examination of the patient to establish the topical location of the lesion. Comparing the symptoms of a local segmental lesion of the SM with the prevalence of conductive, motor and sensory disorders, the nature of changes in the functions of the pelvic organs usually helps to establish the localization of the pathological focus and its volume [62; p. 28-29].

Radiological imaging techniques are currently leading the way in the detection of CNS malformations, including those of the spinal cord and spine. Computed tomography (CT) is one of the most important techniques for neuroimaging the bony component of spinal cord and spine malformations because of its relative accessibility and high informative value. However, radiation exposure and the need for contrast agents limit the indications for this examination in pediatric neurosurgical practice (V.N. Kornienko, N.N. Pronin, 2006). The sensitivity of CT-visualization of neural tissue structures is 29.41% for spinal hernias, 68.42% for lipomas, 11.21% for short terminal filaments; 45.21% for diastematomyelia; 11.11% for dermal sinus. The specificity of this method for the above malformations of the spinal cord and spine is 100%. The sensitivity of CT-visualization of bone tissue structures is 100% for spinal hernias and 100% for diastematomyelia; specificity is 100% for spinal hernias and 100% for diastematomyelia [5; pp. 3-24, 193; pp.493-496].

MRI has led the way in the diagnosis of spinal malformations in recent decades. This is due to the advantages of the method, such as high tissue contrast and resolution, speed of imaging, safety and the ability to obtain real-time information on almost the entire length of the brain and spinal cord and spine. The presence of skin stigmata in the lumbosacral region, the appearance and progression of neurological symptoms, orthopaedic and neurological disorders determine the indications for an MRI examination to search for hidden spinal dysraphism. The sensitivity and specificity of the method for visualising neural tissue structures in selected malformations is 62.5% to 100%. MRI can visualise the cerebral and bony components of malformations of the caudal spinal cord and spine with high informative power for neural and bone tissue [14; pp.413-415, 34; pp.3-24]. In 5.6% of children with SMH, abnormal structures such as hydromyelia, diastematomyelia, and syringomyelia may be cranial to the hernia. Cartilaginous and bony outgrowths may depart from the affected vertebral bodies. Lipomas, dermoid cysts, and teratomas are sometimes found here, compressing the brain tissue. The sensitivity of MRI imaging of neural tissue structures is 100% for spinal hernias; lipomas 73.33%, short terminal filament 62.5%; diastematomyelia 92.85%; dermal sinus 77.77%; specificity is 100% for spinal hernias; lipomas 94.28%, short terminal filament 100%; diastematomyelia 100%; dermal sinus 100%. The sensitivity of MRI imaging of bone tissue structures is 96.55% in spinal hernias; diastematomyelia, 78.57%; specificity up to 100% [5; pp. 3-24, 89; pp. 348-353].

Magnetic resonance imaging (MPT) is the most informative method to diagnose the disease in its early stages and to determine the surgical treatment and outcome (75,129). The capabilities of one-stage imaging of the brain and spinal cord allow the assessment of abnormal drainage function of the cerebrospinal system at the level of the cranio-vertebral junction, and in the brain. MRI can also be used to diagnose other changes in the spinal cord itself such as lipomas and intramedullary cavities (30; pp. 395, 34; pp. 3-24).

The introduction of neurosonography (NUS) into neurological and neurosurgical practice has expanded its wide application in various pathologies of the nervous system: inflammatory diseases, birth trauma, and anomalies of the nervous system [25; pp.201-202; 42; p.324]. The intrauterine diagnosis of pathological changes characteristic of nervous system anomalies is based on the visualization of pathological changes in the spinal cord, pathognomonic signs of hindbrain injury. [20; pp.45-47,125; pp.993-1004].

The NSG visualizes various changes in brain structures, hydrocephalus, hypoplasia of the corpus callosum, and hypoplasia of the cerebellum. This study is generally available and screening for the detection of SPSM in newborns and infants[25; p.201-202]. The location of the lesion and the functional state of the SM structures are determined using such electrophysiological methods as electroneuromyography and registration of evoked electrical potentials of the SM [73; pp. 45-63, 45; p.324].

Comprehensive examination of patients with spinal dysraphia and fixed spinal cord allows the diagnosis of gross extraneural malformations in 18-20% of patients. Malformations of the internal organs in combination with malformations of the central nervous system, affect almost all systems of the body. Abnormalities of the musculoskeletal system accounted for 42%, of the urogenital system, 16-30.5%; of the digestive organs, 27%; of the SCS, 24.7%. In 5-8% of patients, neural malformations are combined with defects of the cardiovascular system (tricuspid valve atresia, unclosed arterial duct, interatrial septal defect) [75; p. 5-24].

In some publications, a high incidence of urinary tract and ano-rectal anomalies in spinal pathology has been reported. Without taking this into account, it is difficult to achieve good treatment outcomes (56; p. 24). Until recently, the diagnosis of bladder dysfunction was applied exclusively to children over 3 years of age, i.e. from the completion of the "mature urinary type". However, there is increasing evidence that this pathological condition also occurs in young children [4; pp. 208, 21; pp. 2-10, 23; pp. 187-194, 60; p. 26]. Early detection of urinary disorders and restoration of normal urodynamics at the level of the lower urinary tract is very important for prevention and timely correction of urinary system lesions. Information about the types of voiding disorders and their treatment in CMH is incomplete and contradictory. Many aspects of spinal pathology are poorly understood. According to Voronov et al. (2011), a unified, comprehensive approach to diagnosis and treatment, the availability of rehabilitation centres, and multifaceted social support for patients with fixed spinal cord syndrome inspire optimism.

§ 1.4. Treatment outcomes for children with spinal malformations

The comprehensive treatment of children with spinal abnormalities remains a complex medical and social problem. The only radical treatment for spinal hernias is surgery. There is still debate about the timing of surgical treatment and the effectiveness of existing techniques. Often, a child with a spinal hernia requires several surgeries to correct related diseases and complications [59; p.41-46]. According to some authors, survival rates of patients with the earliest possible surgical intervention, regardless of the initial prognosis, have improved significantly. Greenberg (2001) recommends that patients with meningomyelocele and meningocele should be operated on within 24-36 hours after birth, and those with lipomyelomeningocele at 2 months or later, depending on the time of diagnosis. Surgical treatment in the hours and weeks after birth prevents complications and promotes better recovery of SM function. [34; c.24]. Intrauterine surgery on over 250 fetuses with spinal hernias in three medical centres worldwide has been shown to reduce hydrocephalus and the indication for bypass surgery from 90% to 50-60% [148, 1 -12].

Survival rates for complex pathologies remain low. According to E.V. Kashin and A.Y. Osin (2008), the direct cause of death in 29.4% of cases is CNS malformations and their complications in 70.6% of cases. In pathomorphological examination, the detection of CNS abnormalities increases by 18.6% and that of concomitant diseases by 34.2%. Children with myelodysplasia have a high degree of disability, which requires finding new ways of improving care. The improvement of the primary neurosurgical stage is considered to be the priority that determines the success of treatment [42; p.324]. After surgical treatment, many authors report pain syndrome regression (88.2%), increased limb strength (60%), improved sensitivity (12.5%), normalization or partial improvement in bladder and rectal function (33.3%) and (41.1%), respectively. At the same time, complications of surgical treatment occurred in 57.6 % of cases as: wound liquorrhea (15.3 %), pseudomeningocele (15.3 %), transient urinary retention (15.3 %); persistent urinary retention requiring bladder catheterization (7.6 %); wound insufficiency (7.6 %); an increase in motor deficit (3.8 %) [59; p.41-46]. Different authors note an unequal degree of damage recovery. Apparently, this is due to differences in the nature and severity of myelodysplasia. The severity of spinal malformations can vary from severe with almost complete loss of CM function to mild, causing no pronounced functional impairment after birth. However, under the influence of secondary causes, both exogenous and endogenous, they form the basis for the occurrence of abnormalities in later life. According to Y. V. Hayduk (2009), early comprehensive surgical and medical correction of spinal malformations, combined with spinal cord damage, can reduce the risk of neurological deficits and improve the quality of life of patients. Recent advances in neurosurgery and related specialties make it possible to remove children with spinal cord and spinal cord abnormalities from the group of "unpromising" patients and improve their social adaptation [33; p.123-125]. A 'secondary spinal cord fixation syndrome' (SCSSS) develops in 10-75% of children after correction of myelomeningocele and lipomyelomeningocele. They subsequently require 'spinal cord release' surgery. Neurosurgical correction is of great importance in the treatment strategy for SPSM. According to leading scientists, microsurgical defixation of the spinal cord should precede orthopaedic and urological interventions [29; pp.53-61, 47; pp.325-326, 90; pp.348-353, 91; pp.119-120]. Many authors report good immediate and long-term results of neurosurgical treatment of SFSM [97; p.28, 98; p.197, 99; p.53-58, 109; p.76-87]. An improvement and stabilization of the neurological status was observed in 75-

100 % of the patients [97; p.28, 98; p.197]. The position on the prophylactic treatment of SFSM remains controversial. Some authors advocate the principle of prophylactic surgical treatment, while others suggest an active-waiting tactic and surgical treatment in case of increasing symptomatology. Some authors point out that treatment courses including medication therapy in combination with therapeutic exercise and massage increase the effectiveness of complex therapy [91; p.119-120].

Chapter summary.

Analysis of the literature has shown that malformations of the SM constitute a significant proportion of spinal pathology in children as isolated anomalies or in combination with other malformations of the spinal cord and/or spine. The publications mainly reflect aspects of diagnosis and surgical treatment of children with spinal hernias or individual anomalies of the spinal cord and spine; the tasks of detecting hidden forms of spinal dysraphism and active treatment of neurological disorders and organ dysfunctions are not adequately reflected. The indications for surgical or complex neurological treatment in individual nosological forms are not clarified; the possibilities of preventing complications that develop in response to surgical interventions for spinal pathology are not studied. There is no analysis of the character and manifestation of pelvic organ dysfunctions, motor, sensory and trophic disorders depending on the type and severity of ostenevular pathology presented by the main nosological form or their presence in coloproctological and urogenital anomalies on the material of one clinic. It follows from analysis of literature that complex treatment of spinal pathology of congenital genesis is aimed not only at providing of cosmetic effect and elimination of particular type of anomaly, but also at correction of other osteoneural anomalies, functional and organic disturbances and related complications. Improvement of the functional status of the organs involved, prevention of secondary complications, and quality of life should be considered the main goals of the comprehensive treatment of children with spinal malformations. However, works on these aspects of a comprehensive approach to diagnosis, treatment, and rehabilitation of children with osteonerval malformations of the spine and spinal cord are scarce.

Chapter II

MATERIAL AND RESEARCH METHODS

§ 2.1. Characteristics of the clinical material

The work is based on an analysis of the diagnosis and treatment outcome of 321 patients: 156 (48.6%) boys and 165 (51.4%) girls, aged between one day and 18 years, with spinal dysraphism of various forms combined with other types of spinal malformations and anomalies of other organs and systems (Figure 2.1).

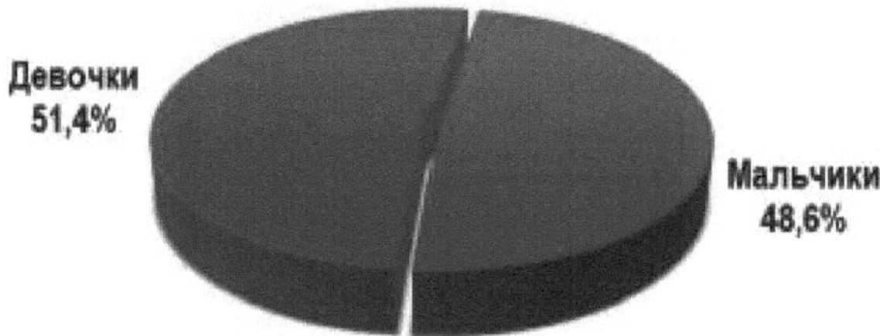

Figure 2.1 Distribution of patients by sex

The patients were treated as inpatients at the routine surgery department of Tashkent City Clinical Hospital No. 2 and at the paediatric neurosurgery department of the Republican Scientific and Practical Centre for Neurosurgery of the Ministry of Health of the Republic of Uzbekistan. They were divided into two groups. The comparison group consisted of 77 (24.0%) patients who were observed in 2000-2011 and examined using the standard diagnostic methods. The main group consisted of 244 (76.0%) patients observed between 2012 and 2016. In this group, spinal pathology was verified taking into account data from functional and instrumental studies: ultrasound, MSCT, MRI of the brain, spinal cord, spinal column; electroneuromyography (ENMG) of the muscles of the lower extremities. Ultrasonography, irrigography, intravenous urography on digital X-ray unit or MSCT were performed to assess anatomical and functional condition of colon and urogenital system. The condition of the vertebrae, structure and location of the spinal cord cone, and terminal filament were assessed, and hidden forms of myelodysplasia were detected. Distribution of patients by sex and age (according to the modified classification of N.P. Gundobin. Tamara Parijskaya, Nina Orlova ; 2017) is presented in Fig. 2.2. and Tab. 2.1

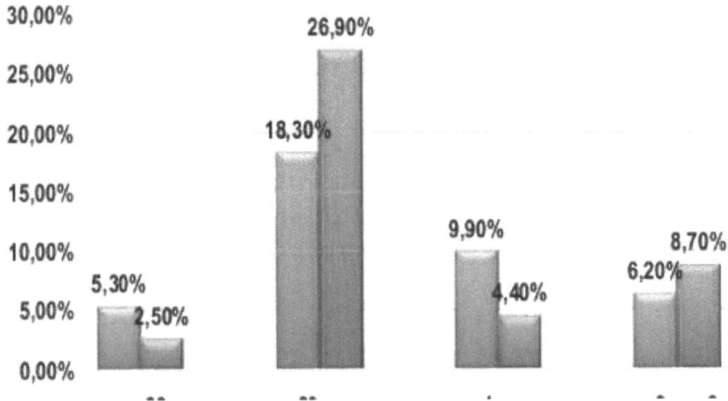

Figure 2.2. Distribution of patients by age and sex

As can be seen from the figure, there were more newborn children and 170 children under 1 year of age (53.0%) among the ill children. Children of preschool age accounted for 14.3%, preschool children 14.9%, primary school children 15.6%, and older school children 2.2%. Since primary school age, there has been a decrease in the frequency of cystic forms with an increase in latent variants of spinal dysraphism.

As shown in Table 2.1, variants of spinal dysraphism were observed in 219(68.2%) patients with different clinical and morphological forms of spina bifida occulta. In 102(31.8%) children spina bifida occulta was associated with: anorectal 51(50%), urogenital 13 (12.75%) anomalies, in 30 (29.41%) with colonic pathology and in 8 (7.84%) in an isolated form. In these patients, there was a combination of osteonervical anomalies in the form of a latent spinal dysraphism leading to functional disorders of the organs concerned (Figure 2.3).

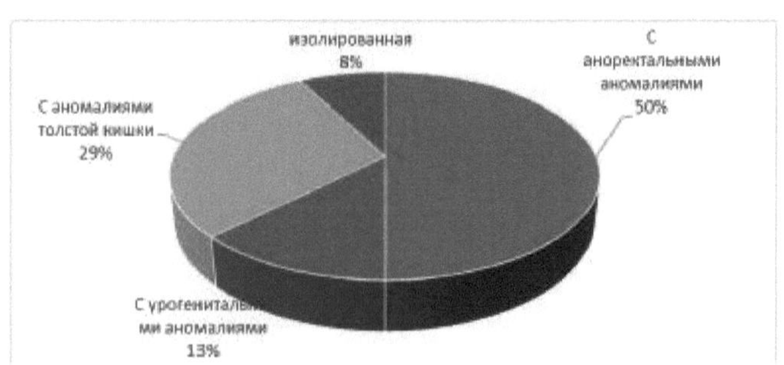

**Fig.2.3 Distribution of patients by form of spinal dysraphism
Spina bifida axulta (n=102)**

Table 2.1

**Distribution of patients by age and form of spinal dysraphism in the main
and comparison groups (n=321)**

Clinical and morphological forms of ostenevular malformations	Age of patients						
	1day-1month.	1 month-1 year	1-3 years	3-6 years old	7-12 years old	13-18 years old	Total
I. Spina bifida aperta (n=219):							
1) Meningocele (n=24)	-/6	3/7	-/3	-/1	-/4	-/-	3/21
2) Meningoradiculocele (n=84):							
(a) Isolated - 31	-/1	9/10	2/3	1/1	2/2	-/-	14/17
b) in combination - 53	-/-	35/-	/-	2/-	8/-	-/-	53/-
3) Meningomyelocele (n=42)	6/7	5/7	2/3	3/3	2/1	½	19/23
4) Myelocystocele (n=8)	-/2	-/5	-/1	-/-	-/-	-/-	-/8
5) Rakhishisis (n=3)	-/2	-/1	-/-	-/-	-/-	-/-	-/3
6) Spina bifida complicate(n=32)	-/-	11/-	2/3	4/-	8/-	4/-	29/3
7) Chiari malformation(n=26)	/-	20/-	4/-	2/-	-/-	-/-	26/-
II.Spina bifida oculta (n= 102):							
1) isolated (n=8)	-/-	2/-	2/-	2/2	-/-	-/-	6/2
2) combined with anomalies other organs (n=94):							
a) with anorectal	1/-	26/-	8/-	10/-	6/-		51

anomalies - 51						/-	-
b) with urogenital abnormalities - 13	-/-	4/-	3/-	4/-	2/-	-/-	13/-
c) with abnormalities of the colon intestines - 30	-/-	-/-	2/-	13/-	15/-		30/-
Total	7 (2,9%) / 18 (23,4%)	115 (47,1%)/ 30 (39%)	33 (13,5%)/ 13 (16,8%)	41 (16,8%)/ 7 (9,1%)	43 (17,6%)/ 7 (9,1%)	5 (2,1%) / 2 (2,6%)	244 (100%) / 77 (100%)

The numerator is the main group and the denominator is the comparison group.

The number of patients by year and form of osteonephritic anomalies in the study and comparison groups was rather uneven (Fig. 2.4). The detection of different types of IDD depended on the leading clinical syndrome and functional features identified by neuroimaging techniques.

Comparison group (2000-2011) n=77

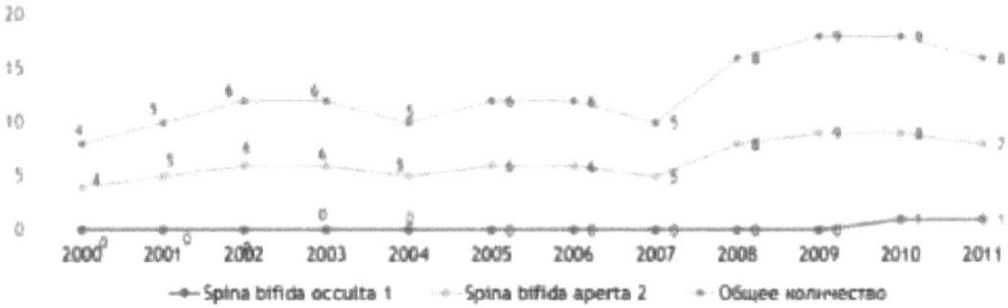

Core group (2012-2016) n=244

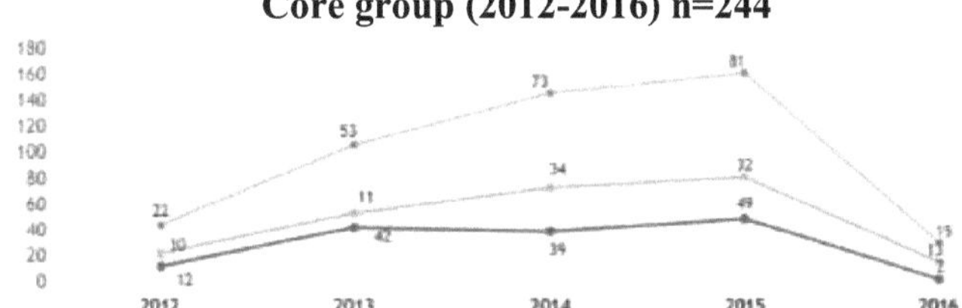

Table 2.2.

Fig.2.4 Distribution of patients by year and form of spinal dysraphism

41

The localisation of spinal dysraphism along the spinal column varied. Irrespective of the type (open or occult), the location in the lumbosacral region was significantly predominant (Fig. 2.5).

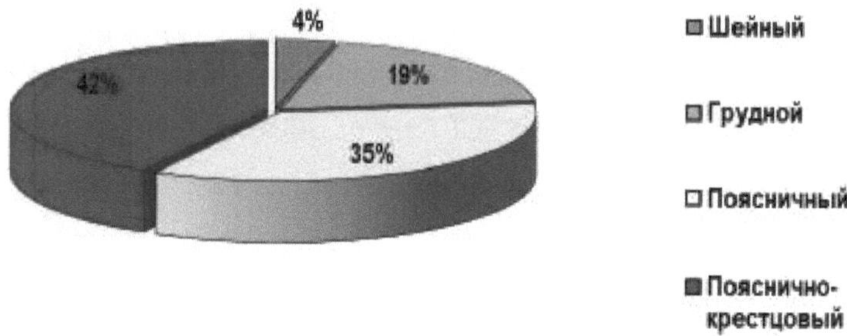

**Figure 2.5. Frequency of localised spinal dysraphism by
to the spinal column**

Of 321 patients with spinal dysraphism, 219 (68.2%) required surgical treatment for cystic forms. Surgeries were performed on 198 (90.4%) patients: 21 (9.6%) (12 patients in the main group, 9 in the control group) due to inoperability (multiple malformations incompatible with life, socially unadaptable complications due to parental refusal) surgical interventions were not performed by collegial decision of doctors of different specialties.

Of 102 patients with occult spinal dysraphism, 94 (92.2%) patients with concomitant anomalies of other organs underwent surgical treatment for established pathology. Surgery was performed at SCDHB No.2 not for spinal pathology but for correction of anorectal, urogenital and colorectal anomalies. Patients of this group required conservative medical and physiotherapeutic treatment for correction of functional disorders caused or aggravated by latent spinal abnormalities 8 children with isolated spina bifida ocularis did not require operative treatment. The presented data indicate that cystic and occult forms of spinal dysraphism are characterized by a high combination of functional abnormalities with anorectal, urogenital and gastrointestinal abnormalities innervated by branches of the most frequently affected lumbosacral region.

Surgical interventions for SMG were carried out mainly at the routine surgery department of Tashkent City CCDB No. 2 - 92 (46.5%) and at the paediatric neurosurgery department of the Republican Scientific and Practical Centre for Children's Neurosurgery of the Ministry of Health of the Republic of Uzbekistan - 96 (48.5%). 10 (5%) children with SMG were operated on in other medical institutions of the country. 161 (81.3%) children with residual phenomena and complications were admitted to specialized departments of SCSD No. 2 (elective surgery, purulent surgery and orthopaedics) for further examination, treatment and rehabilitation with the participation of a neurologist, children's surgeon, urologist and orthopaedist.

94 (92,2%) children with concomitant anomalies of other organs and systems were included in the group of 102 (31,8%) patients with spinal dysraphism due to the fact that in recent years, there was a marked increase in the number of patients admitted to pediatric surgery with anorectal, urogenital anomalies and congenital colonic malformations requiring surgical correction. After surgical treatment at complex examination at them motility disorders of large intestine and functional violations from pelvic organs at normal and satisfactory anatomic structure were revealed. Some patients had no or only low postoperative positive effect after surgical treatment. This has prompted surgeons to investigate children with these pathologies to identify concomitant spinal pathology in order to determine the appropriate treatment in conjunction with a neurologist.

Targeted studies on the causes of unsatisfactory treatment results (clinical and neurological manifestations of a residual nature, trophic disorders and functional disorders in the zone of segmental innervation of the spinal cord) showed the importance of primary examination to identify the combined latent forms of myelodysplasia in the genesis of these disorders. A comprehensive examination of patients with anorectal, urogenital, and colorectal anomalies also showed their high concomitance with latent spinal dysraphism. The predominance of spinal anomalies in the form of lumbosacral dysraphism on the background of rare variants of spinal malformation was characteristic of patients in this group. Verification of the types of spinal pathology proper was performed taking into account the clinical and neurological status and the results, instrumental (ultrasound, MSCT, MRI, EMG) and special urological and proctological methods in SMG (Table 2.2) and anorectal, urogenital and colorectal anomalies (Table 2.3).

Table 2.2

Types of combined latent forms of myelodysplasia and spinal dysraphism in CMH (n=219)

Types of osteonephric malformation disorder	abs.	%
Types of myelodysplasia:		
(a) hydromyelia	18	5,1
b) syringomyelia	17	4,9
c) diastematomyelia	15	4,3
d) pinal lipoma	18	5,1
e) tethering - syndrome	25	7,1
Vertebral anomalies		
Anomalies of the vertebral arches: (a) Defects b) splitting	63 156	18,0 44,6
Vertebral disc abnormalities	2	0,6
Laterolisthesis	2	0,6
Dilation of the spinal canal	4	1,1
Abnormalities in the spine		
Disordered posture: (a) Scoliosis b) kyphosis c) complex deformities (kyphosis + scoliosis)	14 3 2	4,0 0,9 0,6
Abnormalities in the development of the sacrum: (a) Dysgenesis d) hemisacrum	3 3	0,9 0,9
Agenesis of the coccyx	5	1,4
Total	350	100

Of the 219 patients with SMH, 79 (36.1%) had combined forms of occult myelodysplasia. In the preoperative period, they were detected in 62 (78.5%) patients in the main group; after surgery, during additional investigations, in 17 (21.5%) patients with progressive residual neurological disorders and pelvic organ dysfunction.

Table 2.3

Combined lumbosacral dysraphism with anorectal dysraphism,

Types of spinal anomaly	For anorectal anomalies (n=51)		For urogenital anomalies (n=13)		In abnormalities of the colon (n=30)		Isolirospina bifida axulta (n=8)	
	abs.	%	abs.	%	abs.	%	abs.	%
Posture disorders (scoliosis, kyphosis, lordosis)	6	10,9	1	7,7	2	6,7		
Non-enlargement of the arches: (a) One vertebra	6	10,9	3	23	8	26,6	1	12,5
b) two	12	21,82	3	23,1	14	46,7	5	62,525
c) more than two	7	12 7	2	15,38		-	2	
Vertebral body anomaly	2	3,64	2	15,38	1	3,3		
Abnormal development of the sacrum (agenesis, dysgenesis, deviation)	4	7,3	1	7,7	2	6,7		
Coccyx anomalies	6	0,9	1	7,7				
Dilation of the spinal canal	-		-					
Hydromelia	-		-					
Syringomyelia	-		-					
Diastematomyelia	-		-					
Tettering is a syndrome	4	7,3			1	3,3		
Terminal filament lipoma	2	3,64	-					
A combination of separate forms of dysraphia	6	10,9			2	6 7		
Total	55	100	13	100	30	100	8	100

Of the 15 patients with combined forms of myelodysplasia in the comparison group, CT and MRI examinations were not performed in 6 (40%) before surgery. Postoperatively, repeat examinations in these patients revealed a variant of spinal cord fixation syndrome due to the progression of neurological symptoms. The findings indicate that a combination of occult forms of myelodysplasia in SMH is seen in the majority of patients, especially those with severe morphological forms of the disease. They are responsible for the development of spinal cord fixation syndrome when the diagnosis is unknown preoperatively and/or "secondary spinal cord fixation" syndrome in the postoperative period due to pathological fixation of the terminal spinal cord. Their origin, primary (congenital) or secondary (acquired after surgery), is difficult to assess and, with alertness and appropriate diagnostic methods, serves as a reserve for improving treatment outcomes.

§ 2.2. Characteristics of research methods

On admission to the clinic, the initial general somatic and neurological status of the patients was assessed by general clinical, neurological and instrumental diagnostic methods. The data obtained were compared with the results of investigations performed at the stages of treatment (at discharge from hospital, 3 and 6 months after discharge, in delayed to 1 year and remote within 1-5 years) in inpatient and outpatient conditions.

General clinical methods included general blood count; general urinalysis and faecal analysis. Blood serum biochemical tests included determination of total protein, serum protein fractions by electrophoresis; bilirubin and its fractions; ALAT and AST activity, α-amylase - by traditional methods used in paediatric practice. Obstetric history was used to study maternal health, pregnancy and childbirth, forms of genital and extragenital pathology.

During the clinical examination of patients with SMH, the general condition was assessed and aggravating factors were taken into account. The localization of the hernial protrusion along the spinal column, its type, size and condition of the hernial membranes were determined; concomitant diseases and malformations of other organs and systems were identified. Physical development was determined by anthropometric data: body weight, height, head and thorax circumference, length and circumference of extremities in symmetrical areas. For comparison, anthropometric indicators of normal newborns and children under one year of age, proposed by M.E. Abdullaeva (2003), were used.

Objective signs characteristic of a particular form of dysraphia were motor, sensory, trophic, veterinary and pelvic organ dysfunctions of varying severity.

Motor disturbances of the lower extremities in children with peripheral reflex arc lesions were assessed using a five-point MRS (Modified Ronkin Scale). Criteria for assessment of limb muscular strength: 5 points - full movement by gravity with maximal external counteraction; 4 points - full movement by gravity with little external counteraction; 3 points - full movement by gravity alone; 2 points - full movement in a plane parallel to the ground (movement without overcoming gravity) at a comfortable position with resting on a slippery surface; 1 point - feeling of tension while trying to move freely.

The location of the spinal lesion was determined by skin sensitivity according to segmental innervation, taking into account CT and MRI examinations of the spine and spinal cord.

Additional urological and proctological examinations were performed to assess the state of pelvic organ function and to determine the type of urinary and defecation dysfunction. To determine the type of bladder dysfunction, the frequency, volume, and daily rhythm of spontaneous urination were studied; the nature of urge and urine secretion, the degree of urine retention when pressing on the bladder and changing the child's body position were taken into account. Bladder capacity was determined using the formula (child's age in years plus 60 ml) and ultrasound. The amount of residual urine was determined by catheterisation after urination, also by ultrasound. Ultrasonography examined renal status and the presence of vesicoureteric reflux at rest and during bladder filling.

The condition of the rectal obturative apparatus was assessed on the basis of clinical examination of the perineum and anus (closed, partially closed, gaping) and the severity of the anal reflex. The clinical and neurological disorders of the defecation act and the functional state of the rectal obturative apparatus were evaluated according to the developed criteria in points.

Children in the comparison group underwent traditional investigations before surgical intervention. In assessing long-term outcomes, this group underwent a study identical to the main group, in which clinical, paraclinical, instrumental and laboratory methods were performed before - and after treatment. MSCT in patients in the main group did not require spondylography.

To determine the nature of morphofunctional abnormalities in patients with osteonerval anomalies of the spine and spinal cord, a set of instrumental and special methods of investigation were used (Table 2.4).

Table 2.4

**Instrumental methods of investigation in
vertebromedullary malformations in patients (n=321)**

Types of study	Core group	Comparison group	Total
Spondylography	-	30	30
Neurosonography	32	26	58
Echography of internal organs	223	42	265
MSCT spondylomyelography	96	25	121
MSCT of the brain	42	1	43
MRI of the brain	53	5	58
MRI spondylomyelography	100	20	120
MSCT spondylomyelography + excretory urography	30	-	30
MSCT spondylomyelography + virtual colonoscopy	22	-	22
Electroneuromyography	63	28	91

Multispiral computed tomography (MSCT) of the spinal column - spondylomeelography were performed on a Brilliance 64 computed tomography scanner from Philips. The method is highly sensitive and informative in detecting bone-containing hidden vertebral anomalies with concomitant urogenital and coloproctological anomalies. To obtain simultaneous information about the spine and concomitant pathology of the kidney and urinary system, 30 patients received intravenous contrast agent (1ml per kg body weight 76% urogafin, verografin, trazograph) 15-20 min before the examination. MSCT of the spine was supplemented with the study of the colon in virtual colonoscopy mode in 22 patients.

Magnetic resonance imaging (MRI) of the spinal column and spinal cord - spondylomielography was the method of choice for cystic forms of spinal dysraphism. MRI of the lumbar and lumbosacral spine and spinal cord was performed in 3 projections - saggital, coronal and transversal in T1, T2 modes. The examination was carried out in the clinic of SALUS VITA - Soglom Khayot LLC and in the Department of Radiological Diagnostics of 2nd Clinic of Tashkent Medical Academy. General anaesthesia was applied to infants and young children to avoid motor artefacts in the images.

Ultrasound investigation of the nervous system in 32 (13.1%) patients and of internal organs in 223 (91%) patients of the main group was performed on ultrasound scanners of different modifications: Aloka SSD - 1400", ALOKA-500, ALOKA-330, FUKUDA-DENSHI UF-5000 manufactured in Japan. Sector, convex and linear sensors operating in frequency range from 3.5 to 7.0 MHz were used.

Electroneuromyographic examination was performed on a Neuron-Spektr 4/VPM computer electroneuromyograph (Neurosoft, Russia). In order to determine the nature of the root lesion and assess the state of the motoneuronal pool of the anterior horns of the spinal cord, 2 nerves of the lower limb were examined: the right and left tibial nerve. Two main ENMG parameters were determined - motor response (M response) and F wave registration - motor neuron excitation (presence of blocks). In order to exclude neural lesion, excitation propagation velocity along the motor fibres (SRVm) was determined, which was not entered into the data processing. The overlap of the lead electrodes and nerve stimulation points are shown in Table 2.5.

Table 2.5

Positioning of the stimulating and withdrawal electrodes

The nerve to be examined	Positioning the stimulating electrodes over the nerve trunks	Positioning the withdrawal electrodes over the muscle
Tibial right	1. Behind the medial ankle 2. Popliteal fossa	Above the thumb abductor muscle (m. abductor hallucis)
Tibial left	1. Behind the medial ankle 2. Popliteal fossa	Above the thumb abductor muscle (m. abductor hallucis)

The skin surface was treated with alcohol before the electrodes were applied. The tests were usually performed for 15 - 30 minutes at a comfortable temperature, lying on the back against a background of medicated sleep.

Disposable self-adhesive withdrawal electrodes were used at a distance of 1.5-2 cm. The active electrode was placed on the motor point of the muscle, the reference electrode on the tendon of this muscle, and the ground electrode was placed on the other limb. Impedance under the electrodes was 5-10 kOhm.

Stimulation was delivered by supramaximal, rectangular pulses with a stimulation duration of 200 μs. (0.2 ms) with a frequency of 1 Hz. The stimulating bipolar electrode was placed in the projection of the nerve innervating the muscle at its most superficial location.

The data were statistically processed on a Pentium-IV personal computer using the Microsoft Office Excel-2013 software package. Methods of variation parametric and non-parametric statistics with the calculation of the arithmetic mean of the studied parameter (M), standard deviation (), standard error of the mean (m), relative values (frequency, %) were used. Statistical significance of the obtained measurements in comparing the mean values was determined by Student's test (t) with the calculation of the probability of error (P) while checking the normality of distribution (kurtosis test) and the equality of the general variance (F - Fisher's test). To assess statistical reliability of the calculated criteria, we used indices and tables of critical values for acceptable levels of significance (P). Four main levels were taken as statistically significant: high - $P<0,001$, average - $P<0,01$, low (marginal) - $P<0,05$, insignificant (not significant) - $P>0,05$.

Statistical significance for qualitative values was calculated using the χ^2 criterion (chi-square) and the z-criterion (Glantz S., 1998) according to the following formula:

$$z = (p_1 - p_2)\sqrt{\frac{n_1 \cdot n_2}{p(1-p) \cdot (n_1 + n_2)}}$$

where $p_1 = \mu_1 / n_1$ and $p_2 = \mu_2 / n_2$ are the compared experimental frequencies, and $p = (\mu_1 + \mu_2)/(n_1 + n_2)$ the average frequency of the trait in both groups.

Chapter III

RESULTS OF OWN RESEARCH

§ 3.1. Frequency and verification of the clinical and morphological forms of vertebromedullary anomalies in children

Various vertebromedullary anomalies in the form of isolated or combined anomalies of the spine and/or spinal cord with manifest or latent manifestations of spinal lesions were verified in 321 patients aged from 1 day to 18 years, taking into account clinical and neurological status and data of functional and instrumental studies. Extremely diverse and polymorphic in their manifestations, they are observed in children of all age groups. As a rule, cystic forms of spinal dysraphism with obvious external manifestations in the majority of cases 137 (62.5%) are detected during neonatal and infant age. The main manifestations of occult spinal dysraphism have been poorly understood, with a lack of vigilance on the part of clinicians and the exclusion of appropriate tests from diagnosis (Table 3.1).

Table 3.1.

Age of patients at diagnosis of osteonephric malformation (n=321)

Age of patients	spina bifida aperta (n=219)		spina bifida axulta (n=102)	
	abs.	%	abs.	%
Before 28 days of life (n=25)	24	11,0	1	1,0**
from 29 days to 1 year (n=145)	113	51,6	32	31,4***
1 to 3 years (n=46)	31	14,2	15	14,7
3 to 7 years old (n=48)	17	7,8	31	30,4***
7 to 11 years old (n=50)	27	12,3	23	22,5*
12 to 18 years old (n=7)	7	3,2	0	-
total	219	100,0	102	100,0
Note:	* - differences relative to comparison group data are significant (* - P<0.05, ** - P<0.01, *** - P<0.001)			

In 102 (31.8%) patients, individual types of occult spinal dysraphism with varying degrees of neurological deficits or functional disorders of the pelvic organs and/or lower extremities were found as competing pathologies in anorectal, urogenital and colorectal anomalies.

As shown in Table 3.1, the main manifestations are spina bifida aperta - cystic forms of SMH 219 (68.2%) and spina bifida occulta - occult spinal dysraphism 102(31.8%) with failure of the vertebral arches mainly of lumbosacral localisation (Fig.3.1).

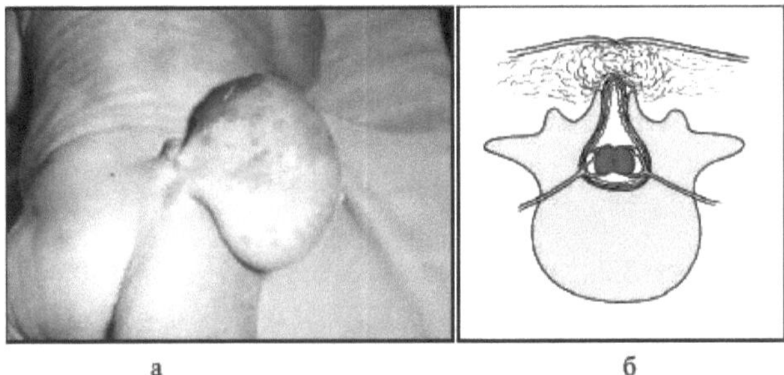

Fig.3.1 Variants of spinal dysraphism: a) spina bifida aperta (patient view); b) spina bifida oculta (diagram).

Osteonephalous malformations of open - 219 (68.2%) or closed - 102 (31.8%) types were presented as: isolated - 148 (46.1%), combined forms with predominance of associated dysraphisms - 79 (24.6%) and in combination with malformations of other organs and systems - 94 (29.3%) (Fig. 3.2).

Careful history taking and clinical examination are important in the postnatal verification of spinal malformations and in the planning of diagnostic and treatment strategies. As a rule, cystic forms of spinal malformations are not difficult to diagnose and are detected by an objective examination of the child. The combination of CMH with lipomatous and teratoid masses and Chiari malformations are also distinguished by characteristic objective features.

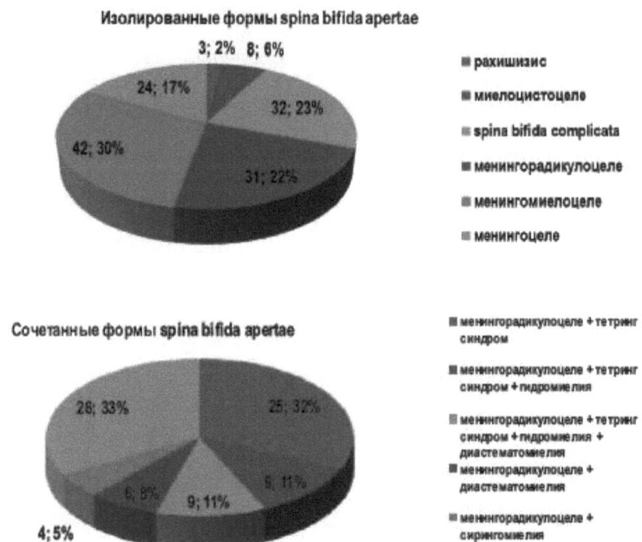

Figure 3.2. Spina bifida aperta (isolated n=140, Combined with ADD n=79)

The presence of cutaneous stigmata of disembryogenesis, motor, sensory, autonomic, trophic, pelvic organ dysfunction, deforming arthrosis without cystic masses alerted us to spinal malformations (Table 3.2).

As can be seen from the table, the main manifestations of spinal dysraphism are spina bifida aperta 219 (68.2%) as a cystic form of spinal hernia (SMH) in 158 (72.0%) of predominantly lumbosacral localisation (62.0%); combination of SMH with teratoid and lipomatous masses - Spina bifida complicate - in 32 (14.6%); Chiari malformation - in 26 (11.9%) and rachyschisis (R) - in 3 (1.4%).

Table 3.2

Clinical manifestations of vertebromedullary anomalies, (n=321)

Clinical and morphological forms of spinal dysraphism	Clinical manifestations						
	Small anomalies (skin stigmas)	Abnormalities of other organs and systems	Motor impairments	Sensory impairment of	Trophic-orthopaedic disorders	Disruption of pelvic organ function	Vegetative disturbances
1.Spina bifida aperta (n= 219)							
(a) Cystic forms n= 158	6	24	144	85	73	116	20

b) Rachyschisis n=3		1	3	3	1	3	2
c) spina bifida complicate n=32	1	3	20	13	4	28	12
d) Chiari malformation n=26	3	4	26	17	9	21	8
2. Spina bifida oculta (n=102)							
(a) Isolated n= 8	-					8	-
b) in combination with abnormalities of other organs (n=94):							
-anorectal anomalies (n=51);	8	14	34	8	-	51	8
-Urogenital anomalies (n=13);		-		3	-	13	6
-colorectal anomalies (n=30)	2	-	10	2	-	30	6
Total	20 (6,2%)	46 (14,3%)	237 (73,8%)	131 (40,8%)	87 (27,1%)	270 (84,1%)	62 (19,3%)

Hidden cleft - Spina bifida oculta - was observed in 94 (92.2%) of 102 (31.8%) patients: in anorectal - in 51 (54.3%), urogenital - in 13 (13.8%) and colorectal - in 30 (31.9%) anomalies accompanied by dysfunction of pelvic organs. In 8(7.8%) patients the pathology was isolated with pelvic organ dysfunction without pelvic organ abnormalities. In diffuse forms of spinal pathology and, in general, spina bifida localisations in the lumbosacral region, anorectal and/or urogenital abnormalities accompanied by pelvic organ dysfunction are often observed. In such cases, in addition to nephrourological and proctological examinations aimed at determining the nature of anatomical-functional, urodynamic and colodynamic abnormalities, patients must be examined for spinal pathology. In order to assess anatomical and functional condition of the colon, urogenital system, and anorectal retention, patients were additionally examined by ultrasound, irrigography, and intravenous urography on digital X-ray unit or MSCT. The clinical presentation and course of myelodysplasia in children depended on the localization and depth of spinal cord root damage, the combination of abnormalities, complications, and the age of the child. The main clinical diagnosis was formulated on the basis of clinical manifestations and data from auxiliary investigation methods. The main significance in the diagnosis of spinal malformations belongs to neurological examination aimed at establishing the topography of spinal cord lesions. Comparison of the symptoms of local segmental spinal cord lesions with the prevalence of conductive motor and sensory abnormalities and the nature of changes in pelvic organ function usually allows us to accurately determine the localization of the pathological focus and its volume.

The pathological process in myelodysplasia is dynamic. The combination of neurological deficits, urological, proctological abnormalities and musculoskeletal deformities is a diagnostic criterion. Cutaneous markers (lipomas, stigmata, dermal sinus, haemangiomas, hypertrichosis and asymmetric buttock folds) were key to recognising spinal dysraphism in 20 (6.3%) patients. One or more cutaneous stigmata in 10 (50%) patients were located in the area of the herniated bulge and in 10(50%) in various areas along the spine (Figure 3.3).

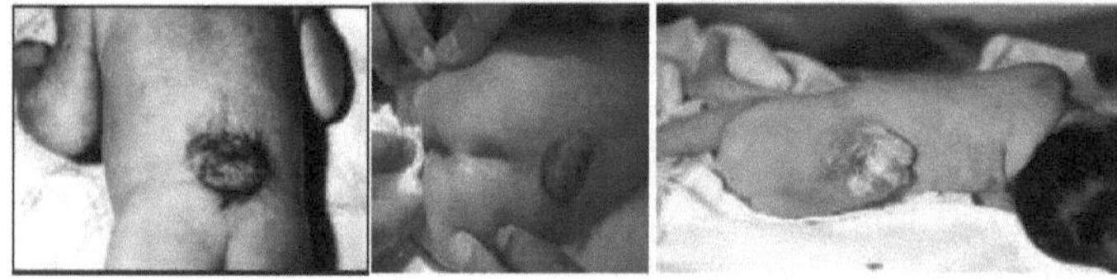

Figure 3.3. Cutaneous stigmata of dysembryogenesis: a) hypertrichosis on the skin of the hernial bulge - patient A, 20 days old, case no. 1245/45; b) pilonidal sinus in the coccyx - patient B., 3 months old, case no. 234/8; c) hemangioma nodules around the hernial bulge - patient B, 3 months old, case no. C., 20 days old, case report no. 453.

On clinical examination, 140 (63.9%) patients were considered to have spinal malformations as an isolated disease. It must be emphasised that the isolation of the malformation is conditional, as other 'invisible abnormalities' may go undetected. It is now recognised that spinal malformations or manifestations of CSD are a marker of potential malformations of the central nervous system and other body systems, requiring examination aimed at detecting concomitant anomalies of the CNS and other organs and systems.

§ 3.2. Diagnosis of osteoneural and spinal malformations in children

In-depth examination according to the diagnostic algorithm developed (Fig. 3.4) made it possible to identify hidden variants of myelodysplasia in CMH (Table 3.3) to identify dysplastic changes on the spinal side - variants of hidden spinal dysraphism (Table 3.4).

As shown in the table, SMH in 140 - (63.9%) patients proceeded as an isolated malformation of the spine and spinal cord. In 79 (36.1%) cases, additional myelodysplasia was detected in separate morphological variants, aggravating the course and outcome of the disease. It should be emphasized that the frequency of these anomalies differed between patients in the study and comparison groups.

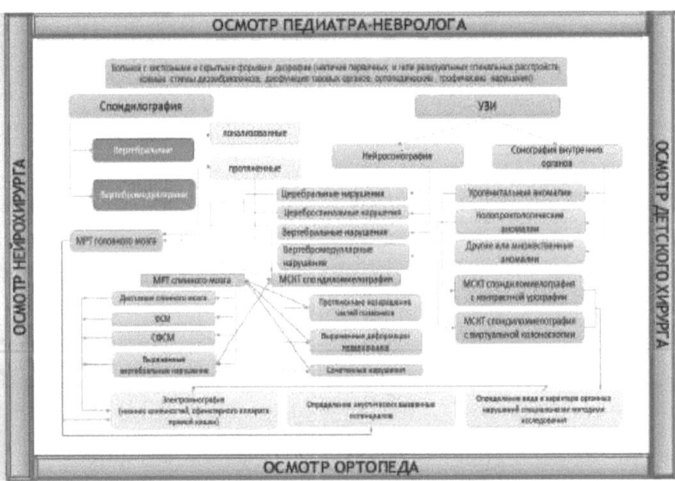

Figure 3.4. Diagnostic algorithm for spinal dysraphia

Table 3.3

Types of myelodysplasia detected by comprehensive examination of patients with cystic spinal dysraphism (n=219)

Clinico morphological forms of SMG	Hydromelia	Diastema tomelia	Siringo-myelia	A combination of several	SFSM	Total
Meningocele n=24						
Meningoradiculocele n=84						
A) isolated n=31						
B) co-mingled n=53	6/3	4/2	4/-	7/-	21/4	44/9
Meningomyelocele n=42						
Myelocystocele n=8						
Rachyschisis n=3						
Spina bifida compli-cate n=32						
Chiari malformation n=26			13/-		13/-	26/-
Total	6 (8,6%)/ 3(33.3%)	6 (8,6%) /2(22,2%)	17 (24,3%) /-	7 (10%) / -	34 (48,5%)/ 4(44,4)%	70 (100%)/9(100%)

Note: Numerator is the main group, denominator is the comparison group.

Of the 15 patients in the comparison group, the combined forms of myelodysplasia were detected in 6 (40%) in the distant period after surgery at the stage of rehabilitation therapy, which is explained by the insufficient amount of preoperative examinations. As the range of special methods of examination in the patients of the main group expanded, the detection of combined anomalies on the part of the spinal cord, spine and other organs and systems increased. The timing of detection and verification of the primary (congenital genesis) and secondary (following surgery for SMG) forms of ASD in patients is of interest, as it determines the plan for surgical tactics and postoperative rehabilitation aimed at the correction of functional and residual disorders (Table 3.4).

Table 3.4

Types of hidden forms of dysraphia detected during surgical treatment in patients in the main and comparison groups

Type of SDS	Total number of	Main group(n=244)		Comparison group(n=77)	
		before surgery	after the operation	before surgery	after the operation
1. In CMH:					
syringomyelia	17	17	-	-	-
diastematomyelia	15	13	-	2	-
SFSM	29	18	5	-	6
hydromyelia	18	15	-	3	-
2. In abnormalities of other organs:					
SSD	91	59	32	-	-
myelodysplasia	7	7	-	-	-
Total	177(100%)	129 (72,9%)	37(21%)	5(2,8%)	6(3,3%)

Spinal malformations were dominated by spinal pathology detected by radiological methods (Table 3.5).

Table 3.5.

Types of spinal anomalies detected in patients with different forms and combinations of spinal dysraphism (n=321)

Types of spinal anomaly	For anorectal anomalies (n = 51)		In urogenital anomalies (п = 13)		In abnormalities of the colon (п =30)		Isolated spina bifida oculta (п = 8)		In CMH (п =219)	
	abs.	%	abs.	%	abs.	%	abs.	%	abs.	%
Posture disorders (scoliosis, kyphosis, lordosis)	6	10,9%	1	7,7	2	**6,7%**			19	5,4
Non-enlargement of the arches:										
(a) One vertebra	6	10,9	3	23	8	26,6	-		36	10,3
b) two	12	21,82	3	23,1	14	46,7	6	75	68	19,4
c) more than two	7	12,7	2	15,38	-		2	25	52	14,85
Vertebral body anomaly	2	3,64	2	15,38	1	3,3			63	18
Abnormal development of the sacrum (agenesis, dysgenesis, deviation)	4	7,3	1	7,7	2	6,7			6	1,71
Coccyx	6	10,9	1	7,7					5	1,43

anomalies										
Dilation of the spinal canal	-		-						4	1,14
Hydromelia	-		-						9	2,6
Syringomyelia	-		-						4	1,14
Diastematomyelia	-		-						6	1,7
Tettering - syndrome	4	7,3			1	3,3			25	7,14
Terminal filament lipoma	2	3,64	-						18	5,14
A combination of individual forms of dysraphia	6	10,9			2	6,7			35	10
Total	55	100%	13	100%	30	100%	8	100%	350	100%

As shown in the table, spinal anomalies of varying severity predominated in 91(92.9%) patients with occult forms of spinal dysraphism combined with anorectal, urogenital or colorectal malformations.

In 33(33.7%) patients with non-marked spinal anomalies (incompleteness of one vertebral arch, moderate scoliosis, hypoplasia of coccyx), functional disorders of the "concerned" organs in the zone of segmental innervation and autonomic disorders were observed. At more rough osteonerval anomalies in 65(66,3%) patients along with the specified disturbances, neurological disorders of various intensity, malformations of urogenital system or coloproctological character were revealed. The high frequency of such combinations indicates the common pathogenetic mechanisms of their development. In such combinations, comprehensive therapy and rehabilitation are required in addition to special investigations. Therefore, the tactics of this category of patients should be determined with the participation of a paediatric surgeon, urologist, orthopaedist, and neurologist.

Spinal malformations are not only characterised by a combination of different osteonephalic anomalies, but also by malformations of other organs and systems that impair the quality of life of the patient (Table 3.6).

As can be seen from the table, the incidence and nature of combined anomalies are varied. The findings indicate the prevalence of concomitant lesions and suggest that congenital spinal anomalies can be classified as multiple malformations.

Table 3.6

Combined malformations of other organs and systems in cystic spinal dysraphism (n=219)

Clinical and morphological forms of osteonerval anomalies	No associated anomalies	CCC	GI	MPS	UDF	Multiple faults	Total
Spina bifida aperta:							
meningocele n=24	24	-	-	-	-	-	24
meningoradiculocele n=84	39	5	4	4	32	-	84
meningomyelocele n=42	23	2	-	-	17	-	42
myelocystocele n=8	-	-	-	-	8	-	8
rachyschisis n=3	1	-	-	-	1	**1**	3
spina bifida complicate n=32	27	-	-	-	5	-	32
Chiari malformation n=26	16				10		26
Spina bifida ossilta:							
isolated n=8	8						8
With anorectal anomalies n=51	42			1	6	**2**	51
With urogenital abnormalities n=13	9			3	1	-	13
With abnormalities of the colon intestine n= 30	28			-	2	-	30
Total	**217 (67,6%)**	**7 (2,2%)**	**4 (1,2%)**	**8 (2,5%)**	**82 (25,5%)**	**3 (1%)**	**321**

The diagnosis of spinal malformations consists of antenatal and early postnatal diagnosis. The diagnosis of neural abnormalities in the foetus in utero is based on the visualisation of abnormal changes in the neural tube and the identification of pathognomonic features. It should be emphasized that throughout the country, despite the sufficient equipment of screening centres for the antenatal detection of congenital anomalies, including neural tube defects using ultrasound, only the presence of spinal dysraphism is noted without analysis and collegial decisions on the management of pregnancy or its premature termination taking into account the severity, operability and possible consequences of the diagnosed anomaly. Such an approach would greatly reduce births with severe forms and complex comorbidities that pose serious problems after birth, or protect pregnant women from unnecessary termination of pregnancy and the birth of a child with a fully correctable anomaly. Thus, antenatal and early postnatal diagnosis of spinal malformations requires increased clinical vigilance on the part of paediatric professionals and targeted examinations in the following circumstances:

- the birth of a child with spinal malformations established antenatally;

- the presence of clear clinical manifestations of cystic CMH in the child;

- Posture disorders and spinal deformities;

- cutaneous stigmata of dysembryogenesis with characteristic localisation along the spinal column;

- urogenital and coloproctological anomalies;

- the presence of asymmetry and trophic phenomena in the lower limb;

- the presence of organic neurological (motor, sensory) symptoms;

- Dysfunction of urination and defecation in the absence of anatomical abnormalities of the pelvic and perineal organs;

- surgical intervention for spinal dysraphism, after which residual phenomena appear or progress.

Chapter summary

The clinical manifestation of spinal malformations occurs in the child at any age. Early manifestation is usually associated with spinal hernias, which constitute the majority of osteonerval anomalies of the spine and spinal cord, occurring in isolation or in combination with other malformations at 219 (68.2%). This group of anomalies is characterized by the presence of latent forms of associated spinal dysplasia, mutually aggravating the severity of the course and neurological consequences in envelope-brain forms of herniation with localization in the lumbosacral spine. According to the localization, nature and severity of dysplasia in the zone of segmental innervation of the spinal cord, neurological, functional disorders of the pelvic organs, probably malformations of the urogenital system and anorectal zone with involvement of the colon sections in the process - 30 (29.4%). The second peak of detection of spinal pathology associated with latent forms of spinal dysraphism occurs at the age of 3-6 years. As a rule, these patients present with urogenital and coloproctological 'involvement', which exacerbates neurological, functional and organ abnormalities.

In myelodysplasia and spinal anomalies, pelvic organ dysfunction, motor, sensory, autonomic and trophic disorders without obvious signs of mental retardation dominate the structure of clinical syndromes. These phenomena persist after surgical treatment for spinal hernia and correction of anorectal, urogenital and coloproctal anomalies. This appears to be due to primary or secondary changes in the spine and/or spinal cord. The presented data indicate the appropriateness of studying the aspects of diagnosis and dynamics of functional and neurological disorders in the stages of treatment of patients with osteonerval anomalies of the spine and spinal cord divided into two groups:

(a) Patients with SMH in isolation - 140 (63.9%) and in combination with occult forms of myelodysplasia - 79 (36.1%);

b) patients - 102 (100%) with latent spinal dysraphism associated with functional disorders and anomalies of the colon, anorectal zone and genitourinary tract.

Chapter IV

CLINICAL AND NEUROLOGICAL CHARACTERISTICS
SPINA BIFIDA APPERTA

§ 4.1. General clinical findings and local manifestations of CMH

Of 321 patients with spinal dysraphism, 219 (68.2%) had spina bifida splitting and cystic hernia formation - spina bifida aperta - as (Fig. 4.1): spina bifida hernia (SMH) - 161 (73.5%); spina bifida complicate (SBC) - combined neural tube formation pathology including different anatomical forms of spina bifida hernia and dystopic lipoma formation, fibrous tissue or with teratoid inclusions of heterogeneous structure around the herniated bulge in cystic cleft - 32(14.6%) Chiari malformation (MC) type 1 and II combined with meningocele or meningomyelocele - 26 (11.9%). Although these nosological forms of spinal dysraphism have their own clinical and anatomical features, what they have in common is the presence of a spinal hernia of different localization and anatomical form.

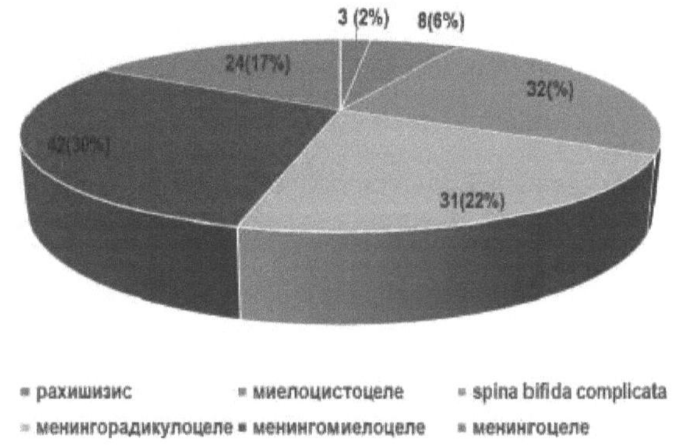

Figure 4.1. Frequency of cystic spinal dysraphism variants

The presence of a spinal hernia is usually established at the initial examination of the neonate. In 219 patients with SMH, the duration of hospital admission for examination, treatment, and assessment of primary neurological status varied (Table 4.1). In the natural course of SMH, the shape and size of the hernial bulge, the condition of the herniation, the severity of clinical manifestations and the complication of myelodysplasia change in the patient.

Table 4.1.

Age of patients with cystic spinal dysraphism at hospitalisation (n=219)

A form of spinal dysraphism	Up to 28th day	From 29 to 1 day	From 1 to 3 years	From 3 to 6	From 7 to 11	From 12 to 18	Total
Spinal hernias (n=161)	6/18	52/30	12/10	6/5	12/7	1/2	36/
Spina bifida com - plicate (n=32)	-	11/-	2/3	4/-	8/-	4/-	29/3
Chiari malformation(n=26)	-/-	20/-	4/-	2/-			26/-
Total	6/18	83/30	18/13	12/5	20/7	5/2	144/75

Note numerator - main group, denominator - comparison group

The majority, 137 (62.6%) of patients were hospitalised before the age of 1 year. Most frequently - during the first month: in the first week - 4 (16.7%), second week - 4 (16.7%), third week - 10 (41.6%), fourth week - 6 (25%) because of such threatening complications as ruptured membranes (4), threat of rupture (6), inflammation of the herniated cover (6), increasing hydrocephalus syndrome (8). When the hernial protrusion was small, there were no hernial complications, and there were no pronounced neurological manifestations, the patients were examined by specialists at different periods of their lives. In these cases, the clinical and neurological status was assessed and treatment tactics were determined during hospital admission. The main reason for the delayed hospitalization of patients older than a year old was the underestimation of a small hernia by medical personnel and parents due to the normal skin. Early identification of the anatomical shape of the SMH and surgical correction are necessary. With delayed treatment, there is a progression of the manifestations of the disease with the onset of various complications. We illustrate a clinical example of a child with a complicated CMH.

The patient Akramova Umida 6 years old, pl. № 5856-334-335 (Fig.4.2) was admitted to the clinic on 01.11.16. The child has been on the "D" registry since birth with the diagnosis "Congenital developmental anomaly, lumbar spinal hernia, hydrocephalus".

Complaints: tumour-like mass in the lumbar spine, limitation of movement in the lower extremities, urinary and stool disorders.

Past medical history: she has been sick since birth. At birth she was diagnosed with CMH and treated conservatively. At home, against the background of a body temperature of 39 g, the child had seizures. The child was hospitalized to Orita No. 2 of Tashkent City CChB.

Somatic status on admission: General condition is severe, with several episodes of seizures.

Locally: a tumour-like mass measuring 9 -10 cm hyperemic in the lumbar region. A yellowish fluid is secreted from the mass.

Neurological status: At the time of examination the child was conscious. In the cranio-cerebral nerves - convergent strabismus, Grefe's symptom + on both sides.Movement in arms is not limited,muscle tone is increased.In legs active movements are limited,muscle tone is increased by spastic type.Muscle strength 2-3 points. Tendon reflexes are elevated D=S, abdominal reflexes are reduced. Pathological reflexes: Babinski, Oppenheim are evoked from 2 sides. Clonus of the foot is evoked on both sides. Pain and tactile sensitivity is preserved. Inflammatory and trophic changes are observed in the lumbar region, around the mass. Pelvic organ function: hyperreflexive type of urinary dysfunction. On ultrasound of the bladder: 10% of bladder capacity. Brain MRI scan: CT scan shows a pattern of occlusive hydrocephalus and intracranial hypertension. Spinal MRI: Abnormal development of the vertebral bodies, Spina bifida on the uroan of the lumbar spine. Meningomyelocele at the level of VL2 to VL3. Signs of diastematomyelia at the level of VL3.

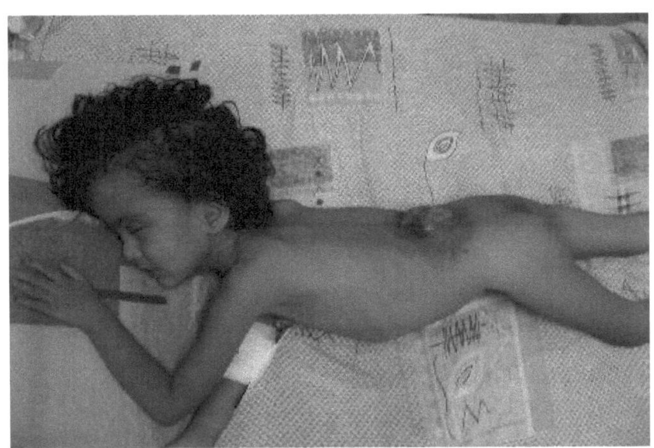

Figure 4.2. Patient A.W. 6 years old. andb #5856-334-335. Complicated myelomeningocele of the lumbar spine.

Clinical diagnosis: Congenital developmental anomaly. Meningomyelocele at VL2 to VL3, diastematomyelia at VL3 with spinal cord dysfunction. An occlusive hydrocephalus. Secondary meningoencephalitis.

Late surgical intervention is indicative of the severity and numerous complications of vertebromedullary complications.

The main determinant of the course, severity of clinical and neurological symptoms, and prognosis of the disease are the anatomical forms of SMH. Of 219 patients, 24 (10.9%) had meningocele, 192 (87.7%) had various envelope-brain forms, and 3 (1.4%) had rachyschisis (Table 4.2).

Table 4.2

Anatomical variants of envelope and envelope-brain forms of herniation in cystic spinal dysraphism (n=219)

The clinical and morphological forms of CMH	LSG (п = 161)		SBC (п = 32)		MK (п =26)	
	Abs.	%	Abs.	%	Abs.	%
1) Meningocele	24	14,9	0	0	0	0
2) Meningoradiculocele	84	52,2	29	90,6	13	50,0
3) Meningomyelocele	42	26	3	9,4	13	50,0

4) Myelocystocele	8	5,0	0	0	0	0
5) Rakhishisis	3	1,9	0	0	0	0
Total	161	73,5	32	14,6	26	11,9

The clinical and neurological status in patients with cystic forms depended on the localisation of the herniated protrusion. Localisation of SMH in the cervico-thoracic vertebrae was observed in 5 (2.3%) patients, in the thoracic in 9 (4.1%), in the lumbar in 76 (34.7%), in the lumbosacral in 92 (42%) and in the sacral in 37 (16.9%) (Table 4.3, Figure 4.3).

Table 4.3

Distribution of patients according to the localisation of a herniated disc in cystic spinal dysraphism (n=219)

Type of dysraphia	Localisation of the hernia									
	In the cervico-thoracic region		In the thoracic region		In the lumbar spine		In the lumbosacral region		In the sacral region	
	abs.	%	abs.	%	abs.	%	abs.	%	abs.	%
Spinal hernias (n=161)	4	80,0	5	55,6	66	86,8	59	64,1	27	73
Spina bifida complicate (n=32)	0	0	2	22,2	3	3,9	21	22,8	6	16,2
Chiari malformation (n=26)	1	20,0	2	22,2	7	9,2	12	13,0	4	10,8
Total	5	2,3	9	4,1	76	34,7	92	42,0	37	16,9

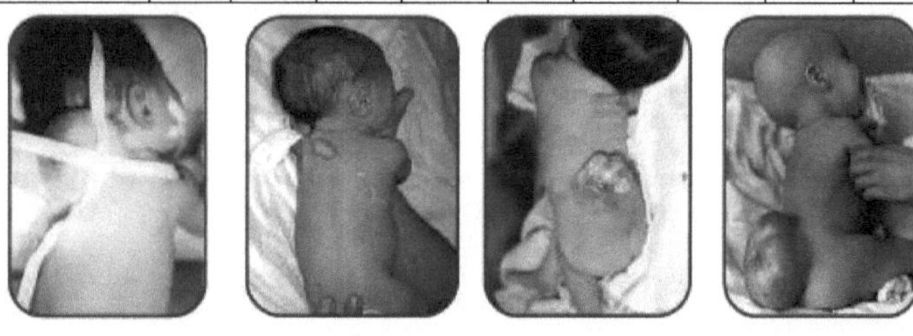

Figure 4.3. Localisation of SMH in different parts of the spinal column: a) cervico-thoracic, b) thoracic, c) lumbar, d) lumbosacral

The size and shape of the herniated bulge also determines the severity of the clinical and neurological symptoms, as the area of the defect along the spinal column varies. The transverse size of the herniated sac ranged from 1.5 to 12 cm.

According to the size, we divided hernias into: small, up to 5 cm in diameter, 88 (40.2%); medium, 5-10 cm in diameter, 104 (47.5%); and large, over 10 cm in diameter, 27 (12.3%) patients. In the globular form, the herniation can involve from 2 to 5-6 vertebrae and occurs as a variant of the envelope-brain form. In the pear-shaped form, the area of the defect is minimal and consists mainly of meningocele (Figure 4.4).

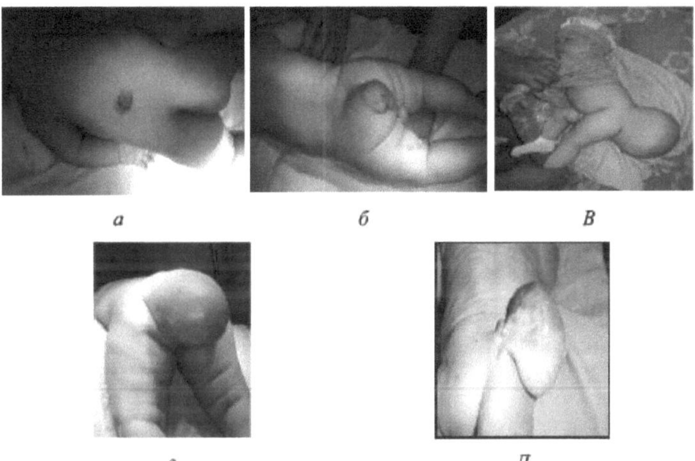

Figure 4.4. Different sizes and shapes of SMG:
a) small; b) medium; c) large d) globular; e) pear-shaped.

The size of the herniation does not always correspond to the nature of the osteonephritic anomaly. In barely noticeable hernias, more extended vertebral clefts are possible (Fig. 4.5).

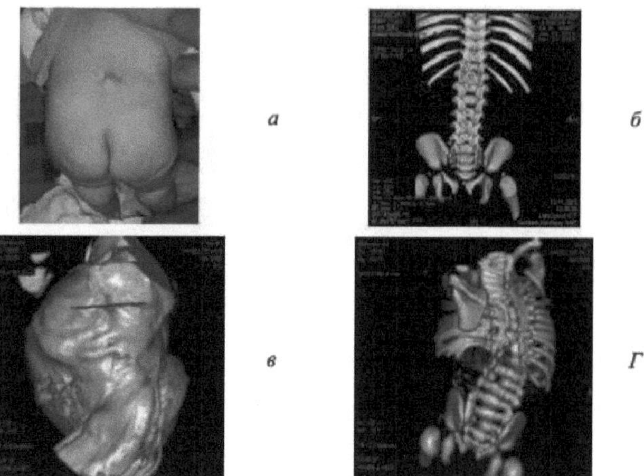

Fig.4.5 Disproportionate hernial bulge size and area split vertebrae:
a) View of a small hernia, b) CT scan of the spinal column of the same child - complete
(d) Lumbar vertebral arches not protruding; patient W. H. H., 3 months old; c) herniated protrusion in the lumbar region; d) CT scan shows complete cleavage of the lumbar and thoracic vertebrae; patient N.S., 6 months old; case #2356-67

The condition of the hernial cover is one of the main factors influencing the course of SMH in children and the occurrence of complications. Of 219 children, 84 (38.4%) had hernias completely covered by normal skin and subcutaneous fat (Fig. 4.5a). In 55 (25.1%) patients the skin over the hernial bulge was thinning towards the apex. In 26 (11.9 %) cases the hernia was covered by thin skin throughout (Fig. 4.6 b). In 22 (10%) patients the thinning skin was intimately fused with the hernia sac. In 12 (5.5 %) children there was rupture of the sheath (Fig. 4.6 c). In 20 (9.1 %) children, purulent or purulent-fibrinous inflammation of the hernia sheath was diagnosed (Fig. 4.7. a).

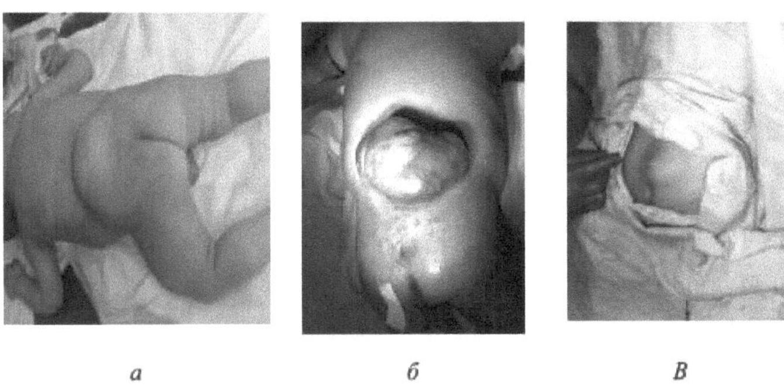

**Figure 4.6. The condition of the hernia cover in SMH:
a) covered with normal skin, b) covered with thin skin,
c) rupture of the membrane with liquorrhoea**

In 6 (30%), there were scarring changes in the hernia sac (Fig. 4.6.b). In the latter three complications, there was a high likelihood of ascending meningoencephalitis and an increasing cerebrospinal hypertension syndrome. These complications occurred in 14 (43.8%) neonates. Concomitant intrauterine infection of the fetus had a significant influence on their occurrence and progression.

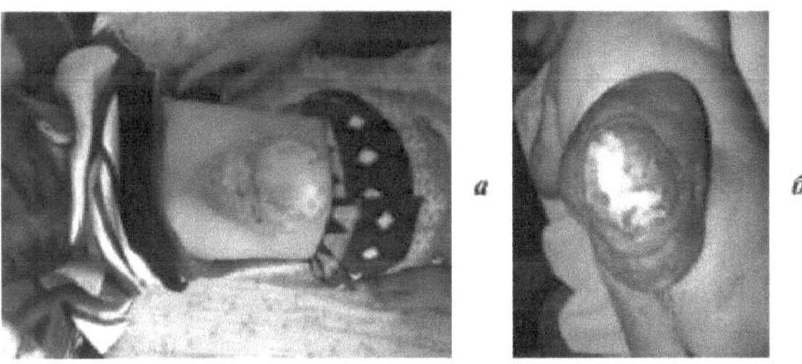

**Figure 4.7. Purulent inflammatory changes of the hernia cover in SMH: a)
scar changes, b) purulent-fibrinous inflammation**

In 12 (37.5%) out of 32 patients, spina bifida complicate was represented by a lipomatous mass enveloping the spinal hernia, localized along the spine, spreading paravertebral, smoothly passing into the subcutaneous tissue. In 17 (53.1%) patients with small hernial protrusion, the mass located along the spine had a round or oval shape. In 3 (9.4%) observations, the lipomatous inclusions were giant, asymmetrically flattened paravertebral to the right and left side, without a clear appearance and transition to the surrounding subcutaneous tissue. Irrespective of the size of the lipomatous inclusion, the lesion was localised in the lumbar region and was covered by normal skin (Fig. 4.8). The paucity of neurological symptoms in these observations was the main reason for the late referral of the patients' parents to a specialist.

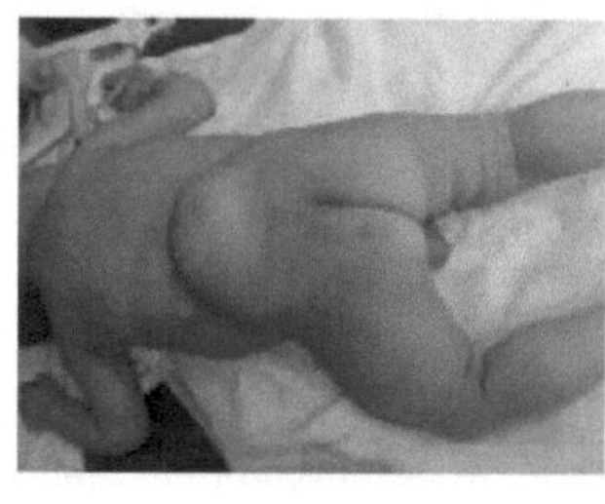
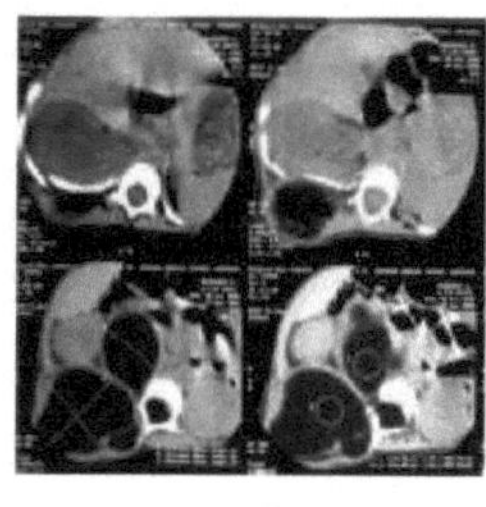

a   *б*

Figure 4.8. Lipomeningocele in the lumbar spine in patient R.H., 1 year 6 months, hist. 681-2.
a) Type of herniated dislocation, b) CT scan of the spine

In subcutaneous localisations of large lipomatous tissue, diagnosis was not difficult. The use of ultrasound allowed the true size of the 'tumour' and the hernia itself to be established and the differential diagnosis of large spinal hernias with a lipomyelomeningocele to be made (Figure 4.9).

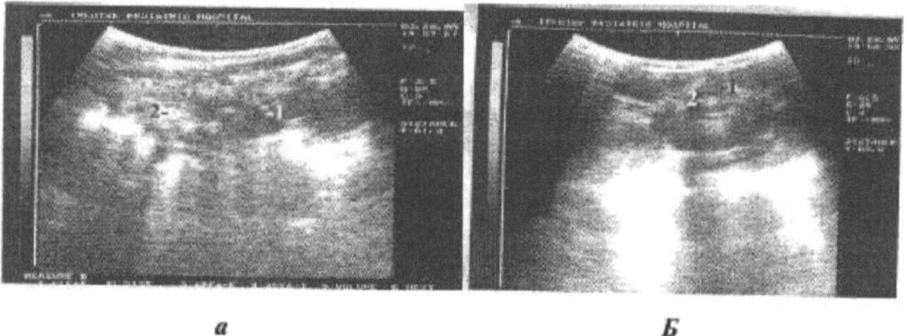

a   *Б*

Figure 4.9. Echograms for lipomyelomeningocele, patient K., 9 years old:
a) axial scan 1 vertebral canal; 2 lipomatous tissue; b) longitudinal scan 1 vertebral canal; 2 lipomatous tissue.

In 12 (37.5%) cases, the structure and localization of a tumor-like mass in the lumbosacral spine was characterized by the fact that, despite the medial location of the tumor-like mass base, its protruding part of heterogeneous density and often with a knobby surface covered by alternating areas of normal and thin skin containing organoid structures, was located to the left or right of the midline, giving an unusual appearance to the hernia. In two cases, a combination of malformations of the spinal cord, spine and dystopian atypical local organoid tissue was observed when the process was localized to the thoracic spine. In one girl, a tumor-like mass measuring 5x6 cm along the spinal column looked like a mammary gland areolae on the background of a pigmented hairy nevus (Fig. 4.10 a). In another patient, a "tumor-like" mass of the same localization appeared as a rudiment of the hand and finger (Fig. 4.10 b).

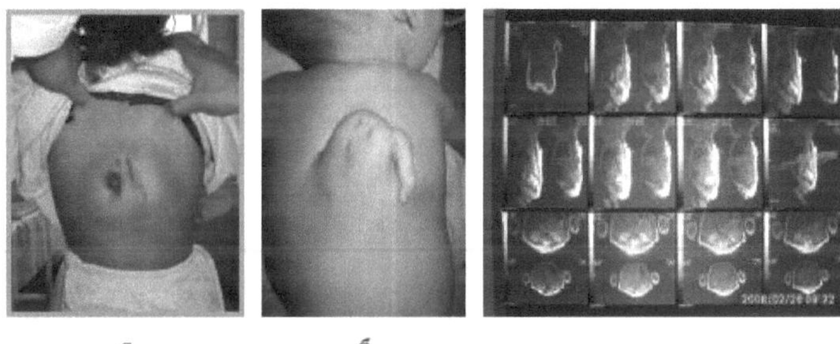

a *б*

**Figure 4.10: b) Spina bifida complicate in the thoracic spine with a teratoid mass: 1) View of the mass, 2) CT scan of the spine -
Patient A.U. age. 3 months old; b) spina bifida complicate in the thoracolumbar spine, patient A. U., age 3 months. U., 3 months old, (O.D. No. 745-208-69): a) teratoid herniated dislocation, b) CT scan of the spinal column - congenital VTh 12-V L1-3 non-dislocation, lipomeningo-radiculocele detected**

In the third child, the case is similarly casuistic. In the lumbar spine, there was a spinal fragment consisting of the buttock and right lower extremity (Fig. 4.11). In all these observations, the pathological masses were directly associated with the spine or spinal cord sheaths - spina bifida complicate. Histological examination showed the presence of ectopic tissue of heterogeneous structure, which was not typical for this localisation, which allowed them to be considered teratoid.

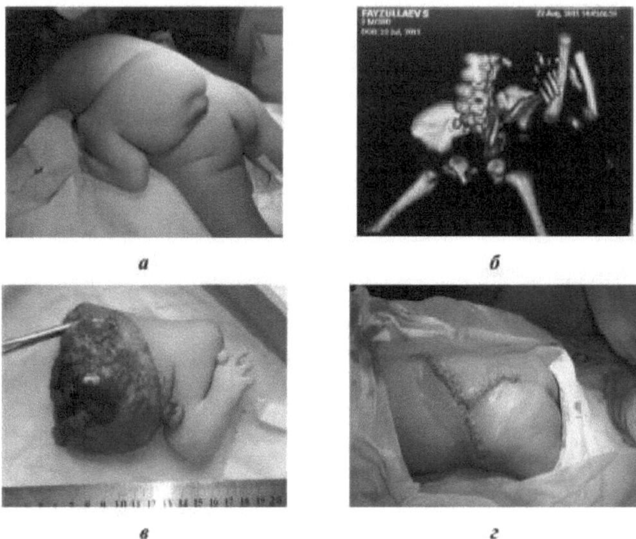

**Fig. 4.11. Spina bifida complicate in the lumbar spine,
patient F.W., 6 months old, (pl. no. 745-208-69):
a) teratoid inclusion consisting of lower limb fragments, b) CT scan of the
vertebral column - deformity and non-overlap VS 1-VS 1U determined, c)
removed macropreparation, d) post-operative view**

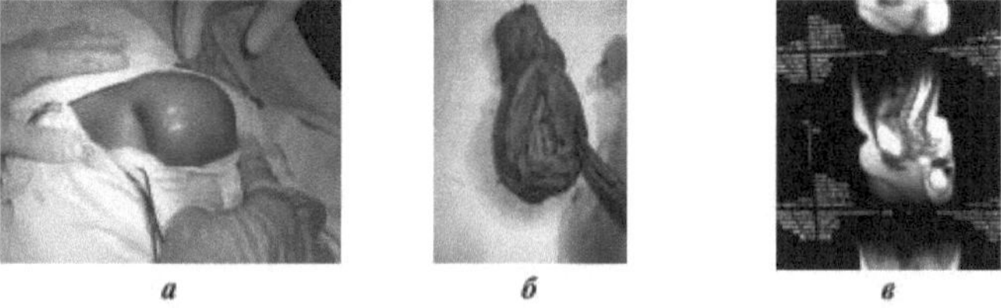

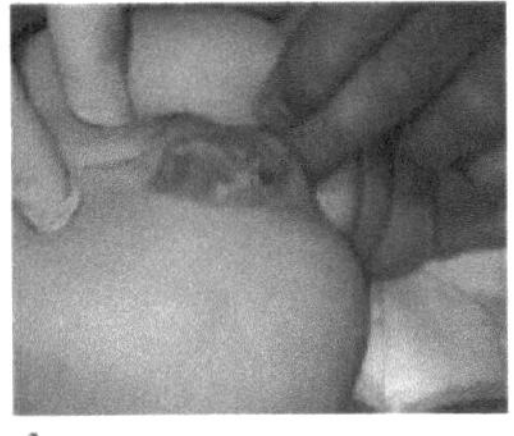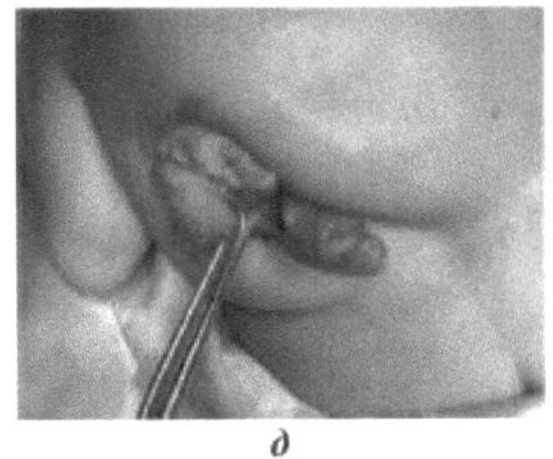

в　　　　　д

Fig. 4.12. Spina bifida complicate asymmetrically located in the sacral spine. patient A. D. 8 months of age (case report 8991-207); a) view of the hernial bulge, b) macro preparations of the removed "tumor" resemble the female external genitalia of girls, c) CT scan of the same patient - the defect area and tumor tissue and connection with the caudal spine are visible, d, e) materials of other operated patients - tissue fragments resembling male and female genitalia are identified in the thickness of the hernial bulge Organs

In Spina bifida complicate, in 3 observations, miniature male or female external genitalia were clearly visible in the thickness and surface of the mass (Fig. 4.12). 17 (7.8%) of the 219 patients with SMH in both groups were born prematurely at 34-36 weeks gestation. Birth weights ranged from 1916 to 4830 g.

At determination of anthropometric data in 71 (32.4%) cases height and weight of a body corresponded to the age indexes; physical development retardation was noted in 136 (62.1%) cases, severe retardation in 8 (3.7%), paratrophy in 4 (1.8%) patients (Figure 4.13).

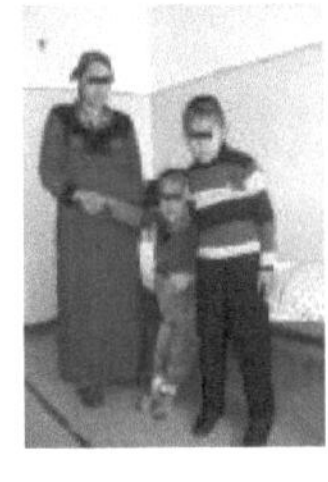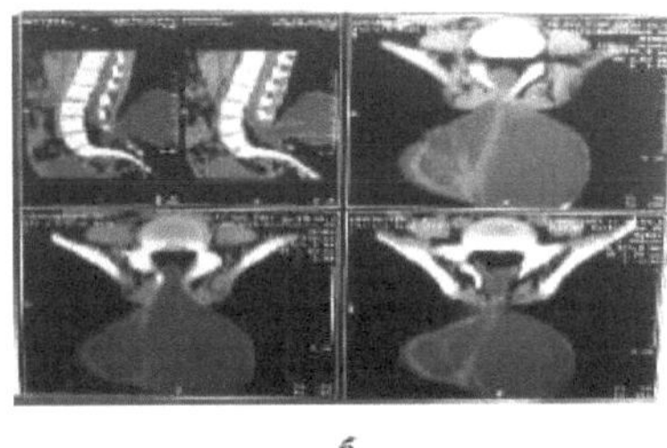

a　　　　　б

Fig. 4.13. Severe developmental delay in CMH, patient X. 7 years old (hist. no. 637- 133):
(a) The photo shows Hasan between his mother and his twin brother Husan;
b) MSCT of the patient's spine - meningoradiculocele in the lumbosacral spine.

The condition of patients (Table 4.4) at the time of admission was of little concern, with the exception of 137 (62.5%) neonates and infants. In 35 of these patients deterioration was due to underlying disease, comorbidities or comorbidities such as intrauterine infection in 12 (10.2%); bronchopneumonia in 11 (7.9%); perinatal lesions of the nervous system in 12 (13.6%).

Table 4.4

Distribution of patients with cystic spinal dysraphism according to severity

Status	Until the 28th day of life	From 28 days to 1 year	From 1 to 3 years	From 3 to 6 years of age	From age 7 to 11	From 12 to 18 years of age	Total abs.	%
Satisfactory	0	66	5	4	4	2	81	37,0
Of medium severity	4	10	25	12	23	5	79	36,1
Heavy	10	35	1	1	-		47	21,5
Extremely difficult	10	2					12	5,5
Total	24	113	31	17	27	7	219	100

In 24 (11%) patients the severity of the condition was exacerbated by complications from the herniated membrane: rupture of the membranes with liquorrhoea in 9 (37.5%), purulent inflammation of the herniated membranes with the development of secondary meningoencephalitis in 15 (62.5%).

§ 4.2. Neurological status and paraclinical findings in cystic spinal dysraphism

In the diagnosis of spinal malformations, in addition to the clinical status, a neurological examination aimed at establishing the nature of the spinal cord lesion is of great importance. Comparison of the symptoms of local segmental lesions of the spinal cord with the prevalence of conductive motor and sensory disorders, the nature of changes in pelvic organ function usually allows the localization of the pathological focus, its volume and characteristic local changes. The clinical manifestations of cystic forms of spinal dysraphism depended on the localisation, size and anatomical variant (Table 4.5).

Table 4.5

Clinical and neurological manifestations in different forms of cystic spinal dysraphism (n=219)

	Clinical and morphological forms of cystic variants of spinal dysraphism	Clinical manifestations							
		Small anomalies (skin	Anomalies of others organs and systems	Motor violations	Violations sensitivity	Trofico-ortho-pedi violations	ities of function Pelvic or-	Vegetative violations	Cranial injury - cerebral nerves
1	Meningocele n=24	-		10/	-	-	-	-	
2	Meningoradiculocele n=84	6	20	84	52	40	66	11	23
3	Meningomyelocele n=42		4	42	25	25	42	6	
4	Myelocystocele n=8			8	8	8	8	3	
5	Rachyschisis n=3		1	3	3	1	3	2	
6	Spina bifida complicate n=32	1	3	20	13	4	28	12	6
7	Chiari malformation n=26	3	4	26	17	9	21	8	20
	Total	10 (4,5%)	32 (14,6%)	193 (88,1%)	118 (53,9%)	87 (39,7%)	168 (76,7%)	42 (19,2%)	49 (22,4%)

The severity of neurological abnormalities in 193 patients with SMH ranged from minor reflex disorders to paralysis. The most severe neurological abnormalities were detected in the postnaroscapular localisation of the pathological process. The following neurological symptoms were seen in patients with the cerebellar form in the lumbar and sacral spine: 16 (8.3%) had increased knee and Achilles reflexes, 177 (91.7%) had these reflexes decreased; 155 (80.3%) had marked paraparesis with impaired pelvic organ function; 38 (19.7%) had paraplegia with impaired pelvic organ function; 118 (61.1%) children had sensory disorders.

Symptoms of insufficient innervation of the cranial nerves in patients with SMH were attributed to concomitant hydrocephalus (48 patients), Chiari malformation (26 patients) and perinatal lesions of the nervous system. Restriction of eyeball mobility was observed in 12 (16.2%) of 74 (33.8%) patients with this pathology, convergent strabismus in 22 (29.7%), smoothing of the nasolabial fold in 6 (8.1%), and decrease of the swallowing reflex and choking when swallowing in 9 (12.2%) patients.

Hydrocephalus was detected in 74 (33.8%) of 219 patients, of whom 26 (35.1%) had Chiari malformation on MRI. In 14 (18.9%) patients, clinical signs of hydrocephalus appeared in the first hours of life and were very pronounced, which facilitated its diagnosis. 42 (56.8%) children before one year of age showed signs of hydrocephalus: tension of the great fontanelle, predominance of the head circumference over the chest circumference, and divergence of the cranial sutures. Progressive hydrocephalus was observed in 18 (24.3%) patients. Progressive hydrocephalus occurred mainly in patients with herniated membranes or very large hernias. Comprehensive medical treatment was effective in children and kept them stable in only 6 (8.1%). Eighteen patients underwent liquor bypass surgery first, followed by surgical treatment of the spinal hernia.

The main clinical manifestations were motor disorders in 193 (88.1%) patients, pelvic dysfunction in 168 (76.7%), sensory disorders in 118 (53.9%), trophic disorders in 87 (39.7%), skin dysembryogenesis stigmas in 10 (4.6%) patients. However, additional investigations were required to clarify the nature of pathology on the spine, spinal cord, other organs and systems, and to understand the nature of polyvalent disorders. Application of the diagnostic algorithm developed by us made it possible to identify hidden variants of myelodysplasia.

Radiation methods have been the main and informative in the diagnosis of vertebromedullary anomalies. The sensitivity and specificity of CT and MRI studies in the detection of spinal malformations are ambiguous in the evaluation of bone and soft tissue masses, including structures of the spinal cord. Computed tomography is a valuable method of imaging bony changes, while MRI is the method of choice in the diagnosis of spinal malformations, associated intravertebral abnormalities and fixed spinal cord syndrome. When the techniques are used simultaneously, their sensitivity and specificity reach up to

100%. According to the results of comprehensive studies, cystic forms of myelodysplasia were found in 140 (63.9%) observations in isolated form and in 79 (36.1%) in combination with latent forms of spinal dysplasia.

The examination has established various variants of osteonephritic anomalies involving structures of the spine and spinal cord: neurospinal dysraphism, pathology associated with changes in the bony structures of the spine - lumbosacral dysraphism. This division is arbitrary, since the presence of one component does not exclude the presence of other components. In 79 (36.1%) patients with cystic variants of spinal dysraphism, myelodysplasia such as hydromyelia, diastematomyelia, syringomyelia, lipomas, and heterogeneous tissues were identified at the level or cranially from the hernia.

The frequency and variants of occult forms of myelodysplasia increased according to the severity of the anatomical variant and the degree of spinal cord involvement. In 18 (22.8%) cases, more than two types of concomitant anomalies were observed simultaneously, exacerbating the severity and course of neurological disorders in the long term.

Table 4.6

Types of myelodysplasia detected in patients with cystic spinal dysraphism (n=219)

Clinico morphological forms of SMG*	Hydromyelia	Diastematomyelia	Syringomyelia	l filament lipoma	of several anoma	SFSM	SWFSM
Meningocele n=24							
Meningoradiculocele n=84	9	6	4		18	11	5
Meningomyelocele n=42	3	2					
Myelocystocele n=8						4	
Rachyschisis n=3							
Spina bifida complicate n=32				18		14	
Chiari			13			13	

malformation n =26							
Total	12 (5,4%)	8 (3,7%)	17 (7,8%)	18 (8,2%)	18 (8,2%)	42 (19,2%)	5 (2,3%)

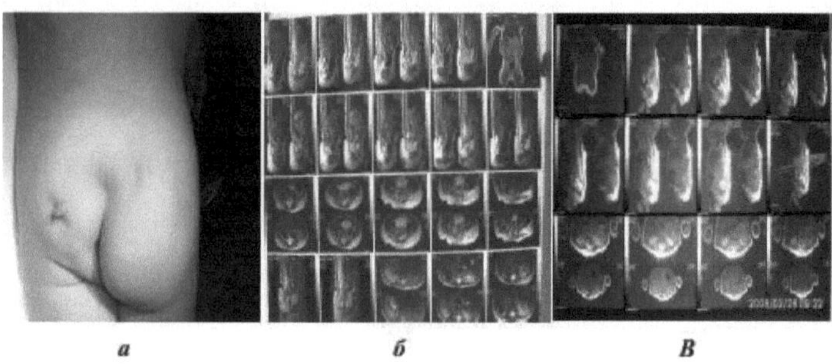

a   б   B

Fig.4.14. Computer tomograms of children with SMH, spinal dysraphism variants: a, b) U. A. 3 y. hist.bol.no.541-1761. tetring - syndrome, hydromyelia L-3-L-4.; c) A. W. 1g. 2m. hist. bol. no. 379-119. diastomyelia, T 11-12-L-1 abnormal vertebrae, diastematomyelia

4.2.1 Musculoskeletal disorders in Spina bifida apperta

Disproportionate growth of the sheaths and spinal cord to the growing spine causes stretching of the nerve fibres, pressing on them by the strained dura mater. Disproportionate muscle traction, trophic effects, aggravating static-dynamic factors, without orthopaedic prevention aggravate deformities of the musculoskeletal system. The severity of movement disorders of the lower extremities in 219 children with cystic spinal dysraphism with lesions of the peripheral part of the reflex arc was assessed using the five-point MRS (Modified Ronkin Scale) (Table 4.7). The localization of the spinal lesion was assessed taking into account cutaneous sensitivity, respectively, segmental innervation, and MRI data of the spine and spinal cord. The nature of symmetry and the type of paralytic deformities of the lower extremities with different localizations were assessed according to generally accepted criteria.

Motor status in children with different variants of cystic dysraphism (n=219)

Clinical and morphological forms of SMG	Assessment of motor status by MRS					Total
	No violations	4 points	3 points	1-2 points	0 points	
Meningocele n=24	14 (58.3%)	10 (41.7%)	-			24
Cerebrospinal forms of CMH n=81 (meningoradiculocele n=31 meningomyelocele n=42 myelocystocele n=8)	-	2 (2.5%)	53 (65.5%)	7 (8.6%)	19 (23.4%)	81
Rachyschisis n=3				-	3 (100%)	3
Spina bifida complicata n=32	12 (37.5%)	4 (12.5%)	16 (50%)	-		32
Meningomyelodiculocele + syringomyelia n=4			4 (100%)			4
Meningoradiculocele + diastematomyelia n=6			4 (66.7%)	2 (33.3%)		6
Meningoradiculocele + hydromyelia n=9			6 (66.7%)	3 (33.3%)		9
Meningoradiculocele + tetring - syndrome + hydromyelia + diastematomyelia n=9			5 (55.6%)		4 (44.4%)	9
Meningoradiculocele + tetring syndrome n=25 A) Meningoradiculocele + spinal lipoma B) Meningoradiculocele + SVFSM		2 (8%)	21 (84%)	2 (8%)		25
Arnold-Chiari malformation (meningomyeloradiculocele + syringomyelia + tetring syndrome) n=26			10 (38.5%)	4 (15.4%)	12 (46.1%)	26
Total	26	18	119	18	38	219

As shown in Table 4.7, motor disturbances were observed in 193 (88.1 %) of 219 patients. On the MRS scale they corresponded to a score of 4 in 18 (9.3 %); 3 in 119 (61.7 %); 1- 2 in 18 (9.3 %); 0 in 38 (19.7 %) children. Impairments were pronounced in severe isolated forms of SMG in 94 (48.7%) children, in combination of SMG with other spinal cord anomalies in 79 (40.9%); in spina bifida complicate in 20 (10.4%) patients. In 164 (85%) patients they were bilateral, in 29 (15%) they were unilateral. Movement disorders were accompanied by other disorders in 87 (45%) of 193 patients: trophic disorders in 30 (34.5%); trophic disorders and joint deformities in 35 (40.2%); joint deformities and trophic ulcers in 22 (25.3%). This can be explained by the fact that severe and combined variants of osteonerval anomaly have increased spinal cord malformations with increasing frequency, variants of their combination with the severity of abnormalities.

The combination of locomotor, trophic disorders with deformity in the joints of the lower extremity indicates the common pathogenetic mechanisms aggravated by associated vertebro-spinal anomalies, which requires early treatment and preventive measures to improve the quality of life of patients. The disorders identified and their combinations depended to a certain extent on the localization and severity of myelodysplasia in the zone of segmental innervation of the spinal cord.

In 57 (26%) of the 193 patients with movement disorders, various deforming arthritis in the joints of the lower limbs was observed, more frequently in the distal direction. Combined deformities of the hip, knee, and foot were observed in 4 (7%) patients; deformities of the buttock were also observed in 4 (7%) cases. Dislocation or subluxation of the hip joint was detected in all these patients. Pathology of the knee joint in the form of flexion contracture between 150° and 90° was found in 2 (3.5%) patients. Paralytic foot deformities of polymorphic nature were detected in 47 (82.5%) patients; in 28 (59.6%) - bilateral with a predominance of equinus component of heel-valgus or flat-valgus deformities. Unilateral pathology was diagnosed in 19 (40.4%) patients (Figure 4.15).

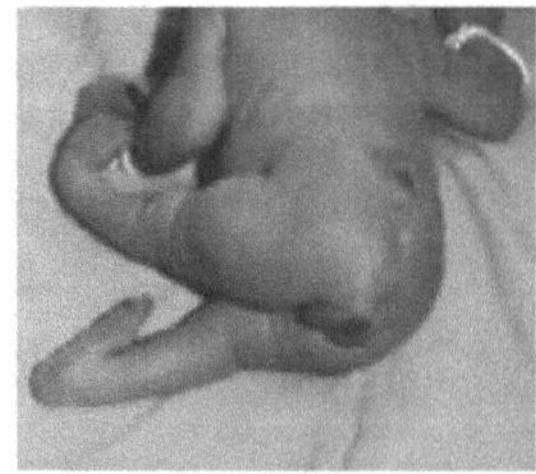 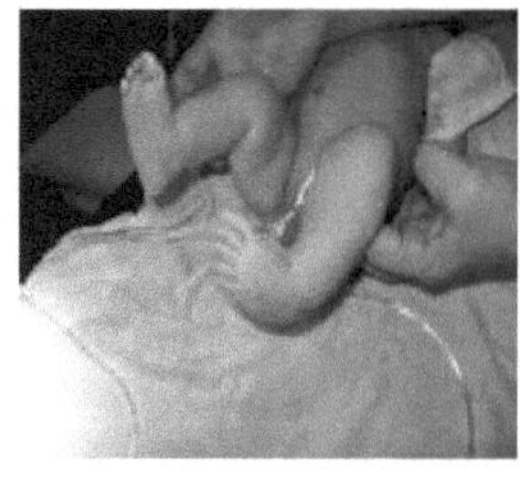

a　　　　　　*б*

Fig. 4.15. obliquity at CMH: (a) on both sides, patient D.N. 1 month old, hist. no. 259; (b) on one side, patient A.R. 1.5 months old, hist. no. №775-272.

Out of 57 patients with different deformities, 24 (42.1%) had movement disorders. In 6 (10.53%) children with lumbar level lesions, subluxation or dislocation of the hip with no arbitrary movements of the lower extremities and wheelchair-assisted mobility was observed due to the absence or weakness of the hip extensor and abductor muscles. 18 (31.58%) patients with severe peripheral paresis (affecting all muscles of the lower extremities with preservation of the knee in some cases and absence of Achilles and plantar reflexes) could stand with support on the knee joints with support on the upper extremities and move around using crutches or other devices. 33 (57.89%) children with different foot deformities walked with a limp.

In severe and extended variants of osteoneural anomaly involving the thoracolumbar spine, 8 (3.6%) out of 219 patients are bedridden and have an imbalance in the proportion of different body regions (Figure 4.16). The data presented indicate that depending on the level and severity of the neurosegmental lesion, as a result of disproportionate muscle traction and force imbalance between muscle groups of antagonists and synergists, statico-dynamic disturbances contribute to the formation of musculoskeletal pathology in the form of deformities in the joints.

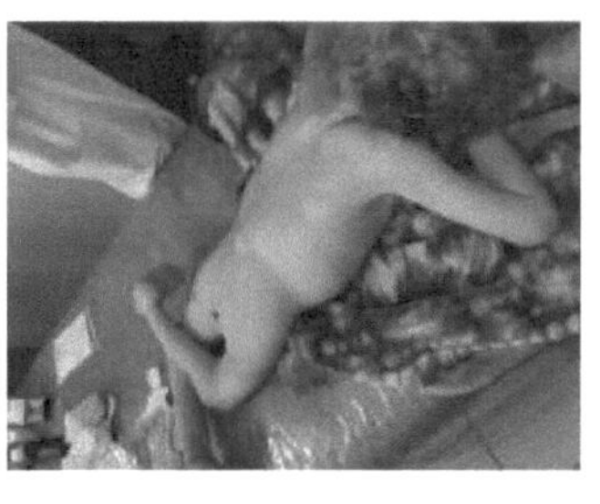
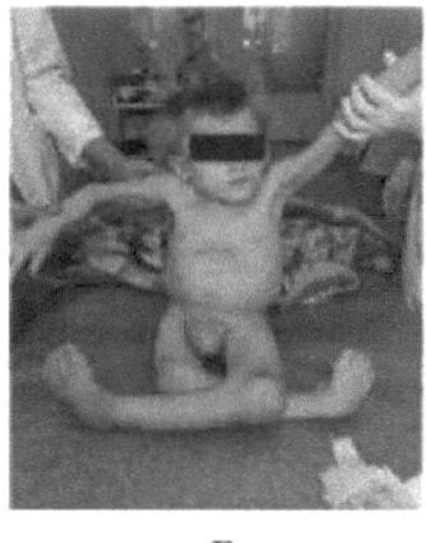

a   *Б*

Figure 4.16. Boln. S.D. 5 years. I/b #345. Disproportion of the different parts of the body with contractures and joint deformities in a combined osteoneural anomaly: a) Rear view; b) Front view.

They result in instability of vertical stability and movement in the lower limbs, which is determined by the specific nature of the damaged area of the nervous system and the area of the body innervated.

Electromyography in 98 (30.5%) patients determined the prevalence of neuromuscular disorders depending on the level of motor segments of the spinal cord. Their topography was determined by comparing the electromyography data and the scheme of segmental innervation of the muscles of the lower extremities, taking into account the proximal border of the spinal cord lesion. As a rule, it was identified by the upper segment innervating the muscles with completely prolapsed function.

4.2.2 Electroneuromyographic characteristics of children with spinal dysraphism

Electroneuromyography (ENMG) is a comprehensive examination of the neuromuscular apparatus, which allows to judge the functional state of the peripheral nerve, the completeness of neuromuscular transmission and the degree of electrical excitability of the muscles. ENMG makes it possible to establish the topicality, acuteness, prevalence and severity of the pathological process in the peripheral nervous system, to trace its dynamics; to differentiate primary muscular diseases; to analyse the effectiveness of the ongoing treatment.

In order to study the nature of the lesion of the p/o roots and the motor neuronal pool of the anterior horns of the spinal cord in children with spinal hernia, as well as to determine the effectiveness of the therapy, we conducted electroneuromyographic studies using the standard technique of stimulation electromyography. All patients of the studied groups underwent electroneuromyography with assessment of the state of sensory and motor fibers, in the formation of which L4, L5 and S1 spinal roots participate, and evaluation of basic neurophysiological indices: amplitude and speed of M-response by motor and sensory fibers of the studied nerves, amplitude and latency of F-wave. Maximum amplitude of sensory response, impulse conduction velocity (ICV) along sensory nerve fibers were recorded. Residual latency, M-response duration, SPI, and F-wave latency were recorded to assess conduction along the motor fibers.

We examined 91 patients with spinal dysraphism aged from 1 month to 7 years. There were 42 (46.1%) boys and 49 (53.9%) girls. The patients were divided into 4 groups according to their age: 2-6 months - 38 patients (41.7%), 7 months-1 year - 16 (17.6%), 1-3 years - 22 (24.2%), 3-7 years - 15 (16.5%) patients.

Patients are divided into two groups according to the nature of the lesion:

- with signs of (presence of) anterior horn motoneuronal pool (MF) lesions (n=41);

- with spinal root lesions without MF lesions (n=50). Electromyographic studies were performed before and after treatment. Control electromyographic studies were performed on 20 healthy children of appropriate age.

To assess the functional state of motor neurons and spinal roots, we included in the analysis the amplitude of motor response from the thumb withdrawal muscle and F wave indices. Here is a brief description of these myographic indices.

The motor response (M muscle response) is the total electrical potential of all the excitable elements of the muscle; it is the electrical equivalent of muscle contraction. The motor response is recorded by indirect percutaneous electrical stimulation of the nerve that innervates the muscle under investigation.

The F wave refers to the late response, which is recorded after the M response. A nerve fibre, as part of a neuron, is an active conductor of electrical potential.

The motor neuronal pool that innervates the muscle has a certain polymorphism. Motor units can be divided into fast (type 1) and slow (type 2) according to their functionality. Slow motor units are less excitable, but can maintain active impulsation for a long time. The axon of these motor units is slow in conductivity. Fast motor units are more excitable, but are quickly depleted by active impulsation. Their axon is rapidly conducting [73; p. 45-63].

From the above, several F-wave parameters are formed that are taken into account in the analysis of neuromuscular pathology.

Given the purpose of our work, we have taken several F-wave parameters that characterise the state of the motoneuronal pool and spinal roots.

The average F-wave latency, a general average characteristic of nerve conduction, is the most stable and is therefore effective for repeated measurements.

Fmax/M amplitude ratio - independent of muscle condition. Reflects to a greater extent the antidromic excitability of the motor neurons. Relatively stable parameter for repeated measurements. Displayed as a percentage

F wave blocks reflect the probability of a minimum ('zero') response when antidromic excitability is reduced. Measured as a percentage.

Average F-wave amplitude - reflects the average amplitude value of the F wave. Depends on the state of the muscle and axonal system. Decreases as conduction slows in the case of increasing desynchronisation of the antidromic response. Measured in µV.

In order to exclude a lesion of the tibial nerve itself, our work also analysed the speed of propagation along the motor fibres of this nerve - srvM. It is measured in m/s.

A correlation between the morphopathology of the spinal cord and roots and the electroneuromyographic findings was made during the analysis of the findings. In spinal root lesions without significant pathology of the motoneuronal pool, the ENMG findings were as follows:

- within the lower limit of normal or a moderate decrease in motor response from the thumb diverter muscle, which averaged 2.8 µV in children from 2 to 6 months and 4.45 µV in children from 7 months to 1 year (73.6% and 76.7%, respectively, of the control group);

- a slight increase in mean F-wave latency, averaging 22.8 ms in children 2-6 months and 25.8 ms in children 7 months to 1 year of age (18.7% and 27.0% respectively from the control group);

- a significant decrease in F-wave amplitude, with an average of 204.3 µV in children 2-6 months and 227.3 in children 7 months-1 year old (56.09% and 49.4% respectively of the control group);

- a significant F-wave block - the average was 63.3% in children aged 2-6 months and 63.05 in children aged 7 months-1 year (8% in the control group).

When the pathological condition involved the motoneuronal pool of the anterior horns of the spinal cord, the ENMG picture changed slightly:

- a pronounced reduction in motor response from the thumb diverter muscle to total absence, averaging 1.0 µV in children aged 2-6 months and 1.8 µV in children aged 7 months-1 year (26.3%, 31.03%, respectively, in the control group). - 1 year old (26.3% and 31.03%, respectively, of the control group);

- pronounced F-wave block up to complete absence (100% block), averaging 87.2% in children 2 - 6 months and 83.6% in children 7 months-1 year (control group 8%);

- increase in Fmax/M-amplitude ratio averaged 4.5% in children aged 2-6 months and 5.15% in children aged 7 months-1 year (69% and 47.14%, respectively, from the control group).

Changes in groups 1-3 years and 3-7 years had the above trend. In children aged 3-7 years without a motor neuronal pool lesion, there were signs of relative muscle reinnervation close to normal. That is, the lowest values were observed in children aged 1 to 6 months with signs of motoneuronal pool lesions. This may be due to immaturity and incomplete differentiation of the motoneuronal pool of the anterior horns of the spinal cord.

In the postoperative period, in 19 (61.29%) of 54 children under 1 year of age, the best results were seen in children with SMG without motor neuronal pool lesions (up to 20.3% improvement from baseline in the early period). When the motoneuronal pool is affected, post-treatment outcomes are modest; more pronounced changes are seen in children operated on early (up to 7.4% improvement from baseline).

In the 1-3 years group, out of 22 patients, 14 (57.14%) and 3-7 years groups, 8 (52.15%) out of 15 patients showed the same trend, with some differences:

- ENMG scores were significantly lower in children aged 1-3 years postoperatively than in children under 1 year of age (up to 15.1% of baseline in SMG without motor neurone damage and up to 5.1% with motor neurone damage);

- children 3 - 7 years old have a sharply increased average Fmax/M ratio (we explain by the fact that over time there is relative reinnervation of the muscles against a relative increase in the functional state of the preserved motoneurons), relatively better postoperatively compared to children 1-3 years old, but lower than in children 0-1 years (up to 17.8 % from baseline in SMG without motoneuron lesions and 5.8 % with motor neuron lesions). We present data before and after treatment (Table 4.8).

Table 4.8

Average ENMG scores in children with SMH with and without motor neuronal pool lesions before and after treatment

Children from 1 to 6 months.	SMH without mot. pool lesions (n=15)		SMH with mot. pool lesions (n=10)		Controle
	before treatment	after	before treatment	After	
Response M amps, mV	2,8±0,30	3,4± 0,32**	1,0±0,27^^^	1,2±0,35^^^	3,8
Cf. lat. F wave, ms	22,8±0,76	22,9±0,28	12,6±2,40^^^	13,5±2,59^^^	19,2
Average blocks by F, %	63,3±4,67	57,6±4,42	87,3±5,62^^	85,2±9,07^^	8
Cfr. Fmax/M r.m.s.a.s. %	4,3±0,87	4,5±0,94	4,5±1,50	4,0±1,27	2,65
Avg. amps. F waves, µV	204,3±21,49	234,1±21,9	167,1±36,59	180,9±39,8	364,2

Children from 7 months Up to 1 year	SMH without mot. pool lesions (n=14)		SMH with mot. pool lesions (n=15)		Controle
	before treatment	after	before treatment	after	
Response M amps, mV	4,5±0,85	5,0±0,86	1,8±0,62^	2,0±0,78^	5,8
Cf. lat. F wave, ms	25,8±0,51	24,6±0,64	13,8±3,54^^	14,2±3,62^^	20,3
Average blocks by F, %	63,0±6,14	53,6±6,24	83,6±5,74^	87,9±4,8^^^	5

Cfr. Fmax/M r.m.s.a.s. %	3,2±0,20	3,2±0,25	5,1±2,37	4,0±1,36	3,5
Avg. amps. F waves, µV	227,3±54,0	262,8±50,3	145,5±41,17	147,8±40,0	459,7

Children from 1-3 years of age	SMH without mot.pool lesions (n=12)		SMH with mot. pool lesions (n=9)		Controle
	before treatment	after	before treatment	after	
Response M amps, mV	2,6±0,52	3,3±0,71	1,8±0,62	2,4±0,78	6,2
Cf. lat. F wave, ms	22,6±1,93	23,4±0,60	15,5±4,49	14,8±4,28^	21,5
Average blocks by F, %	66,0±7,55	66,2±8,71	64,2±18,12	59,5±16,95	4
Cfr. Fmax/M r.m.s.a.s. %	7,5±2,70	8,2±2,43	7,7±3,20	6,2±2,47	3,2
Avg. amps. F waves, µV	221,8±40,7	269,4±38,02	220,8±63,38	222,6±63,71	465,7

Children 3-7 years old	SMH without mot.pool lesions (n=9)		SMH with mot. pool lesions(n=7)		Controle
	before treatment	after	before treatment	After	
Response M amps, mV	5,1±1,10	5,8±0,88	2,6±0,88	2,9±0,88^	7,8
Cf. lat. F wave, ms	24,8±1,60	23,6±0,77	23,2±0,8^^^	22,9±0,48	22,6
Average blocks by F, %	53,1±11,88	33,9±1,03	78,1±4,4^^^	76,3±5,0^^^	2
Cfr. Fmax/M r.m.s.a.s. %	3,5±0,02	3,5±0,15	21,7±0,55	20,4±0,4^^^	3,4
Avg. amps. F waves, µV	167,0±5,50	181,5±4,0*	357,0±17,5	359±19^^^	487,3

Note: * - differences relative to the pre-treatment group are significant (* - P<0.05, ** - P<0.01), * - differences relative to the SMG group without lesions are significant (^ - P<0.05, ^^^ - P<0.01, ^^^^ - P<0.001)

We conclude with the following conclusion.

ENMG studies make it possible to assess the functional state of the spinal cord structures in children with spinal cord and spinal cord abnormalities; the study allows the exact degree of involvement in the pathological process of the spinal roots or the spinal cord itself with the phenomena of compression or irritation of these structures. Changes in ENMG parameters do not always depend on the extent and level of the malformation, but the most significant abnormalities were registered when compressed structures of the spinal cord were involved. Thus, ENMG should be included in the diagnosis of congenital malformations of the spine and spinal cord, in addition to radiological methods, which is important for prognosis and preoperative planning.

4.2.3. Trophic disorders in spinal dysraphism

Trophic disorders of the lower extremities were detected in 87 (45.1%) out of 193 patients with CMH and movement disorders. In 30 (34.5%) patients with trophic disorders, objective examination showed cooling and dry skin with deformation of some toes, thickening of nail plates on the affected side compared to proximal areas and the opposite limb, which was considered to be early vegetotrophic manifestations. In 18 (20.7%) of 87 patients with trophic disorders, marked chromata, a pronounced shortening of the length and circumference of the lower limbs in the form of hypotrophy or atrophy with vegetative-trophic manifestations of an asymmetrical nature were noted: on both sides - in 12 (66.7%), on one side - in 6 (33.3%) patients (Figure 4.17).

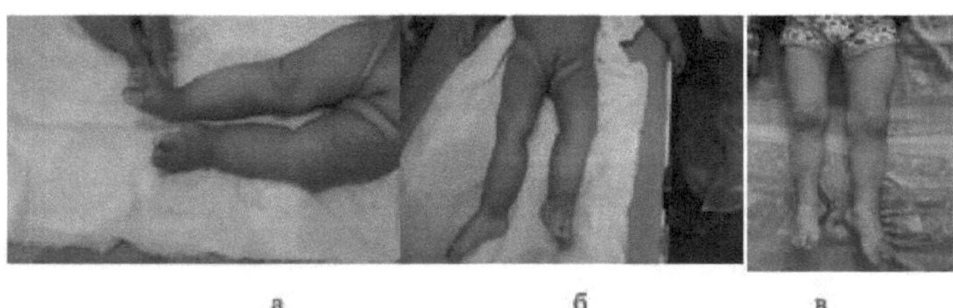

Fig. 4.17. Non-symmetrical atrophy of the lower limbs in SMH:
a-b) bol. N.S. 5 months old bol. no. 790-281-37;
c) patient H. C. 8 years old, hist. ill. no. 2691/628.

In 69 (79.3%) children, a slight asymmetry of the lower extremities due to hypoplasia of the thigh or lower leg muscles was detected. Structural abnormalities of a vegetotrophic nature caused by varying degrees of involvement of the spinal cord structures in the pathological process persist in the form of residual condition in the long term after surgery.

A severe consequence of CMH is a trophic disorder leading to trophic ulcers. The occurrence of this complication in 22 (10%) patients was most frequently observed in severe forms of SMH: meningomyelocele in 12, meningomyeloradiculocele in 7, myelocystocele in 2, rachyschisis in 1 patient. In 14 (63.6%) cases, it was observed in the combined types of occult dysraphism and spinal cord with phenomena of primary or secondary tetring syndrome.

When trophic ulcers were formed, paralytic foot deformities (equinus position, heel valgus, flat valgus) were pronounced. The history revealed that the age of the trophic-necrotic lesions ranged from a few months to years 8 from the onset of the disease or after surgery for CMH. It should be emphasised that none of the cases were alerted to the possibility of this complication and, accordingly, no prophylactic measures were taken.

Unilateral lesions occurred in 10 (45.5%) and bilateral in 12 (55.5%) cases. In bilateral lesions, the size, localization, depth and shape of trophic manifestations on both limbs were asymmetrical, and the affected area showed signs of trophic disorders from the initial stages to ulcer formation. More pronounced disorders were observed on the affected side, where the phenomena of limb atrophy and deformity in the joints were distinct and persistent. The heterogeneity of sensory and motor disturbances in the affected and contralateral limb in the unilateral, or both limbs, in bilateral localization of trophic disorders or ulcers can be explained by the different involvement in the pathological process of radicular structures on the right or left, the degree and the extent of the spinal cord damage.

A trophic ulcer can form on any area of the body where there is prolonged tissue contact with an object that causes compression or microcirculatory disturbances. In 7 (31.8%) patients there was a single localisation of the process, and in 15 (68.2%) there was multiple localisation (Fig. 4.18). In all cases there was involvement of the foot, plantar surface, heel area, 1 or 5 toes, where microcirculatory disturbance occurs more frequently and more intensively.

Trophic ulcers were of different shapes: round - 3 (13.6%); oval - 4 (18.2%); irregular - 15 (68.2%); their sizes varied from 2.0×2.0 cm to 2.0×4.0 cm.

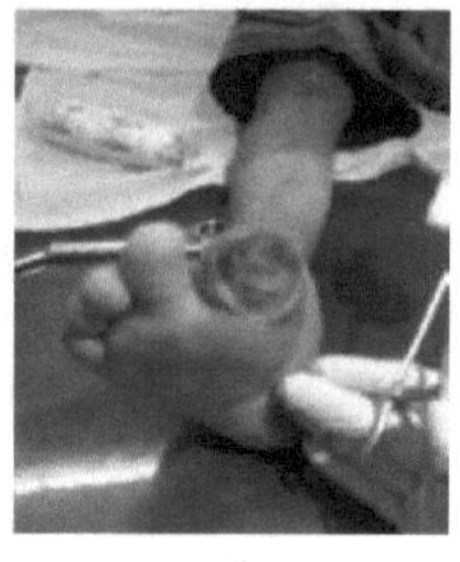
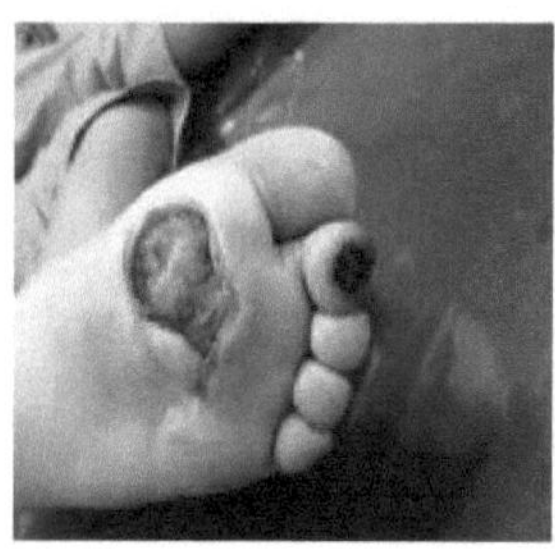

a   Б

Fig. 4.18. Single (a) and multiple (b) trophic ulcers in a spinal dysraphism patient A.N., age 8. 8 years old. hist. no. 4567/34

As the disease progresses, the shape of the ulcers changes and their area increases. With prolonged disease and without adequate treatment, trophic ulcers can grow to enormous sizes.

Pain in the area of the trophic ulcer is moderate or absent. This is due to decreased sensitivity in the affected area. Patients therefore present late, when the ulcer increases in size and pain occurs, usually associated with an outbreak of infection and inflammation in the surrounding tissue, with the development of a purulent-destructive process characterised by a long course, sluggish healing and a tendency to relapse. In the long-term course of the process, the purulent-destructive phenomena deepen with transition to bone tissue - trophic osteomyelitis, which occurred in 2 of our observations (Fig. 4.19).

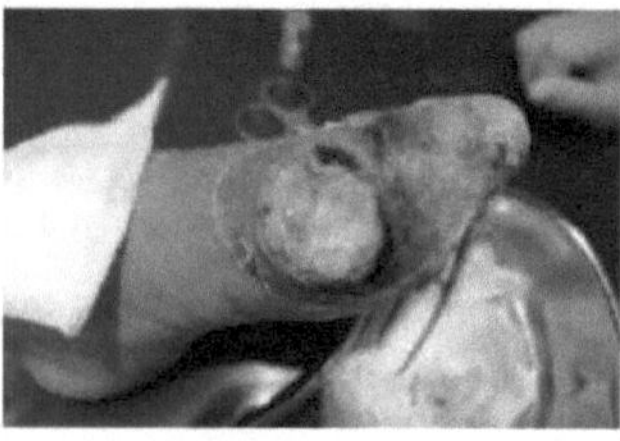
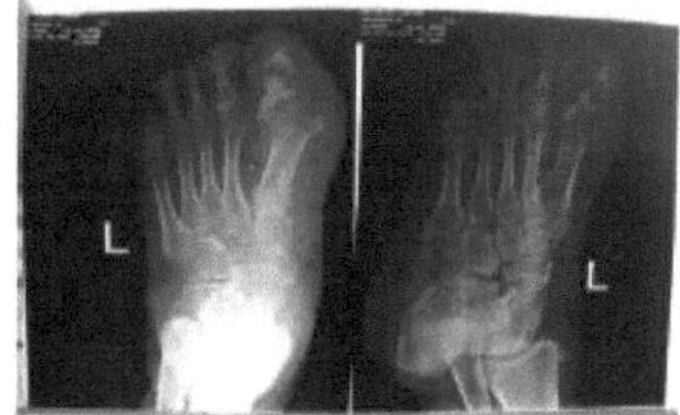

Fig. 4.19. Trophic ulcer complicated by osteomyelitis of the nail phalanx and metatarsal bone of the 1st toe of the left foot. P.G. 13 years old, and/b. №2778-439

When the bone tissue is affected, the process takes a protracted course, and the effects of chronic purulent intoxication and concomitant diseases are markedly intensified. One patient operated on for SMH, with concomitant bilateral ureterohydronephrosis transformed into secondary renal shrinkage with the development of urosepsis, died.

Any additional pathological process contributing to trophic and microcirculatory disorders is an aggravating factor in the rapid development of destructive changes, leading to life-threatening consequences.

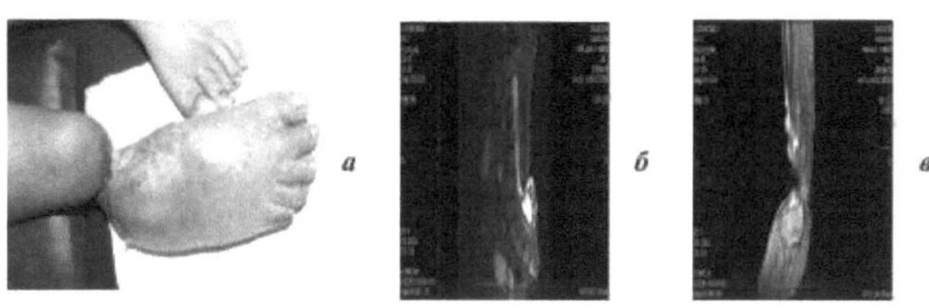

Fig. 4.20. View of the lower third of the tibia and left foot with signs of trophic disorders and ulceration in the presence of amniotic retention (a), spinal CT scan - tethering syndrome (b), CT scan of the lower leg and foot - soft tissue and bone thinning of the lower leg; patient B., 18 years old, hist. №.1353-216-99-245

A 17-year-old girl with myelocystocele in SMH, who was not operated on due to inoperable pathology, had multiple trophic disorders of the lower extremities, which were complicated by the development of necrosis of the foot (Fig. 4.20) and required amputation of the lower third of the tibia.

The presented evidence shows that trophic ulcers are one of the severe complications of severe forms of spinal pathology aggravating the course of the disease and social disadaptation of the patient. Depending on localization and the degree of involvement of spinal structures trophic disorders can transform into single or multiple ulcers of different size and depth with predominant localization in the distal parts of the lower limbs. Trophic ulcers are chronic and recurrent, with a tendency to increase in size and deep tissue involvement, irrespective of the cause. In such cases, the involvement of various specialists is necessary.

4.2.4 Pelvic organ dysfunction in children with myelodysplasia and combinations of osteonephritic pathology with coloproctological and urogenital abnormalities

Pelvic organ dysfunction in the form of voiding and defecation are common clinical manifestations of vertebromedullary anomalies. Pelvic organ dysfunction is common in cystic variants and occult spinal dysraphism, often determines the degree of adaptation of the patient, and is of greater concern to parents than other manifestations of the disease. Of 321 patients with neurospinal dysraphism, 270 (84.1%) had pelvic organ dysfunction: 168 (62.2%) with spina bifida aperta; 102 (37.8%) with spina bifida occulta.

Pelvic organ dysfunction was determined by a general clinical examination, neurological examination and paraclinical examination. The nature and severity of the voiding and defecation disorders were assessed according to the established criteria and the results of special investigations. Contrast MSCT examinations of the colon and urinary tract were additionally performed to detect anatomical abnormalities.

In 168 (62.2%) patients, isolated or combined types of pelvic organ dysfunction were due to spinal malformations proper.In 102 (37.8%) patients, these dysfunctions occurred in latent spinal dysraphism combined with anorectal, urogenital and coloproctological abnormalities. The main manifestations were constipation, faecal incontinence, incontinence or urinary retention alone or in combination (Table 4.9).

The severity and type of dysfunction differed according to the nature of myelodysplasia, localisation and area of cleavage. In cystic forms of spinal dysraphism, pelvic dysfunction was observed in 21 (12.5%) meningoradiculocele, 42 (25%) meningomyelocele, 28 (16.6%) spina bifida complicate, 66 (39.3%) meningomyelocele with additional forms of occult myelodysplasia, rachisis in 3 (1.8%) patients.

Table 4.9

Pelvic organ dysfunction depending on the nature of the underlying pathology (n=270)

Type of violation	Nature of pathology									
	SMG, n=168		Anorektal anomalies with SSD, n=51		Urogenytal anomalies with SSD, n=13		Colorectal anomalies with SSD, n=30		Isolated SSD, n=8	
	abs.	%	abs.	%	abs.	%	abs.	%	abs.	%
Core group										
Chronic constipation	5	4,3	8	15,7	0	0	14	46,7	0	0
Chronic constipation with paradoxical fecal incontinence	5	4,3	12	23,5	0	0	2	6,7	0	0
Fecal incontinence	1	0,9	16	31,4	0	0	0	0	0	0
Urinary incontinence	62	53,0	5	9,8	10	75,9	1	3,3	4	66,7
Urinary retention	2	1,7	0	0	0	0	0	0	0	0
Chronic constipation and incontinence	4	3,4	6	11,8	0	0	8	26,7	0	0
Fecal matter and urine	38	32,5*	4	7,8	3	23,1	5	16,7	2	33,3*
Total	117	53,9	51	23,5	13	6,0	30	13,8	6	2,8
Comparison group										
Chronic constipation	4	7,8	0	0	0	0	0	0	0	0
Chronic constipation with paradoxical fecal incontinence	0	0	0	0	0	0	0	0	0	0
Fecal incontinence	1	2	0	0	0	0	0	0	0	0
Urinary incontinence	20	39,2	0	0	0	0	0	0	0	0
Urinary retention	0	0	0	0	0	0	0	0	0	0
Chronic constipation and incontinence	0	0	0	0	0	0	0	0	0	0
Fecal matter and urine	26	51,0	0	0	0	0	0	0	2	100,0
Total	51	96,2	0	0	0	0	0	0	2	3,8

Note: Numerator is the main group, denominator is the comparison group. * - Differences relative to the comparison group are insignificant (P>0.05)

95

In latent spinal dysraphism, splitting within a single vertebra at the S1 level was observed in 17 (16.7%); splitting of two or more vertebrae in 46 (45%); splitting of vertebral bodies in 5 (4.9%); anomalies of the sacrum in 7 (6.9%); splitting of vertebral bodies in combination with malformation of coccyx - in 7 (6.9%); complex, combined forms of occult spinal dysraphism - in 15 (14.7%); posture disorders (scoliosis, kyphosis) - in 9 (8.8%) patients. In this group of patients there are concomitant abnormalities of the genitourinary system and coloproctological organs, accompanied by a disturbance of the anatomical structure, which negatively affects their functional state.

General clinical and neurological examination, evaluation of bladder sonography data (frequency, rhythm of urination, bladder volume in the accumulation and emptying phase, the child's urinary retention capacity) and other investigations were the basis for verifying the following urinary disorders in 84 (38.7%) of 217 children in the main group with pelvic disorder.

The hyperreflexive type was found in 39 (46.4%) patients. It is characterised by urge: often imperative; increased frequency of urination exceeding the age norm by 3-4 urinations; decreased volume of urine, prolonged urination despite small amount of urine; decreased age-specific effective bladder volume, presence of residual urine over 10% of the bladder capacity.

A hyporeflexive type of disturbance was found in 19 (22.6%) patients with characteristically decreased urination; often the act of urination is performed by pressing the parents on the bladder. Detrusor volume is greater than that of the age group. Detrusor threshold sensitivity to changes in bladder volume is reduced. Dripage of urine when the bladder is full, flow increases with pressure on the bladder and change of body position. Incontinence during stress conditions (crying or laughing, straining, coughing), residual urine over 30% of the bladder capacity.

Detrusor-sphincter dyssynergy in 26 (31%) patients showed bladder contraction aimed at emptying the bladder; the sphincter acts in the opposite direction, trying to prevent this act. This type of bladder dysfunction often goes unrecognised due to similarities with the hyperreflexive type of disorder. The urge in these children is often imperative and the urination is more frequent with less urine. There is an intermittent flow of urine. In some patients the act of urination stops when the bladder is pressed. Residual urine is more than 20% of the detrusor capacity.

To determine the nature of the defecation disorder, the state of the rectal obturator was assessed by clinical examination, and the state of the perineum and anus (closed, partially closed, or gaping) was determined by the severity of the anal reflex. The anus is normally closed. A tonic contraction of the muscles of the voluntary sphincter accompanied by retraction of the anus when the skin on the inner thighs or around the anus is irritated shows that the anal reflex is completely intact. In severe disorders of the innervation of the pelvic floor and perineum, there is no retraction of the anus when stimulated, appearing sagging, in the form of a 'perineal hernia'.

Isolated defecation was found in 63 (29.0%) out of 217 patients in the main group with pelvic disorders. The defecation disorder was observed in the form of chronic constipation in 27 (42.8%) patients; in 28 patients it was combined with urinary dysfunction. Constipation combined with paradoxical incontinence was observed in 19 (30.2%) patients, in 26 patients it was combined with urinary dysfunction. Anal sphincter insufficiency with faecal incontinence isolated - in 17 (27%) patients (in 16 combined with urinary dysfunction). Chronic constipation in myelodysplasia may be due to colosfincter dyssynergy due to pelvic diaphragm rigidity, which is inadequately involved in reflex activity of colon emptying; impaired innervation of abdominal muscles due to lesions of sympathetic and parasympathetic innervation zones or distal spinal cord. The anus is tight, the abdominal, anal and Achilles reflexes are reduced, and there may be difficulties in voluntarily increasing the anal sphincter tone during rectal examination, in which patients may experience a delay of 3 to 4 days of independent stools. These children are given purging enemas or laxatives for bowel emptying.

In chronic constipation with paradoxical faecal incontinence, defecation is absent or infrequent. Fecal stones form due to an accumulation of faeces. These children usually have intermittent faecal stools due to impaired innervation of the sphincters of the rectum.

Grade I anal sphincter insufficiency with fecal incontinence in 11 patients showed a regular sense of urge and physiological act of defecation, with involuntary small portions of faeces being excreted occasionally. In grade II (5 children), there is still a sense of defecation, with occasional conscious defecation. However, more or less faeces are excreted involuntarily every day. The perineum and buttocks are constantly stained with faeces, the skin around the anus is irritated, and there is an unpleasant odour, to which others react negatively. The child has to be cleaned several times a day and his underwear has to be changed. In stage III 1 patients, there is no sense of urgency and no conscious defecation and there is a constant, involuntary excretion of faecal material.

The results of the examination show that children with CMH, in addition to paralysis and paresis, have marked somatic diseases. In connection with pelvic organ dysfunction, pyelonephritis, chronic renal failure, intestinal dysbacteriosis and hypotrophy are detected.

4.2.5 Sensory disturbances in Spina bifida aperta

Among the neurological manifestations of osteneural anomalies of the spine and spinal cord, sensory disturbances are a significant feature. In 216 children under 3 years of age, pain sensitivity was investigated; from 3 to 7 years, tactile and pain sensitivity was assessed (48 children). In 57 children 7 years and older, superficial and deep sensitivity was assessed (Table 4.10).

Table 4. 10

Sensory disorders in spinal dysraphism as a function of patient age (n= 321)

Sensory impairments	Age						Total	
	1 day to 1 month.	1 month to 1 year	1 year - up to 3 years	3 - 7 years	7- 12 years old	12 years and over		
No dropouts - 2	5	75	16	22	26	4	148	60,7%

98

points	7	21	6	4	4	-	42	54,5%
Hypoesthesia - 1	-	23	16	18	17	1	75	30,7%
point	6	8	3	3	2	2	24	31,2%
Anaesthesia - 0	2	17	1	1	-	-	21	8,6%
points	5	1	4	-	1-		11	14,3%
Total	7	115	33	41	43	5	244	100%
	18	30	13	7	7	2	77	100%

Sensory disorders were observed in 131 (40.8%) out of 321 patients. Depending on the localization of the lesion and the degree of involvement of spinal structures, sensory disorders manifested as segmental, radicular changes in the form of hypoesthesia, anaesthesia on the lower limbs and perineum of varying severity in cystic forms in 118 (53.9%) and latent spinal dysraphism in 13 (12.7%) patients.

Of 219 patients with spina bifida aperta, 101 (46.1%) had no sensory disturbances. Hypoesthesia and anaesthesia were found in 118 (53.9%) (Table 4.11). Sensitivity disorders were manifested by segmental, radicular changes in the form of hypoesthesia on the perineum and lower extremities. The examination of deep sensitivity clarified the child's ability to understand what was required of him or her. The severity of hypoesthesia and anaesthesia of the lower extremities (more often the sole and posterior surface of the tibia) was symmetrical in most cases in 117 (89.3%) children. Right-sided was recorded in 6(4.6%) patients, left-sided in 8 (6.1%). Hypoesthesia and anaesthesia in the anogenital region was noted in 47 (35.9%) patients, indicating involvement of the spinal cord cone.

Table 4.11

Condition of sensitivity depending on the type of cystic spinal dysraphism of patients in the main group (n=144) and the group comparison (n=75)

Clinical and morphological forms of spinal pathology	No violations		Hypesthesia		Anaesthesia		Total (abs/%)
	OH	HS	OH	HS	OH	HS	
Isolated forms							
Meningocele n=24	3	21	-	-	-	-	3(2,1%) 21(28%)
Meningoradiculocele	7	9	4	7	3	1	14(9,7%)

99

n=31							**17(22,7%)**
Meningomyelocele n=42	7	10	8	12	4	1	**19(13,2%)** / **23(30,7%)**
Myelocystocele n=8	-	-	-	5	-	3	**0** / **8(10,7%)**
Rachyschisis n=3	-	-	-	-	-	3	**0** / **3 (3,9%)**
Spina bifida complicate n=32	19	-	7	-	3	3	**29(20,1%)** / **3(4%)**
Meningoradiculocele + tetring - syndrome n=25	7	-	12	-	6	-	**25(17,4%)** / **0**
Meningoradiculocele+ diastematomyelia n=6	4	-	2	-	-	-	**6(4,2%)** / **0**
Meningoradiculocele+hyd e-romyelia, tetring - syn-drome n=9	3	-	6	-	-	-	**9(6,3%)** / **0**
Meningoradiculocele + hydro-myelia + diastematomyelia, tetring - syndrome n=9	2	-	6	-	1	-	**9(6,3%)** / **0**
Meningoradiculocele + syringomyelia n=4	-	-	-	-	4	-	**4(2,8%)** / **0**
MC*+ meningoradiculocele +syringomyelia, tetring - syndrome n=13	4	-	9	-	-	-	**13(9%)** / **0**
MC*+meningoradiculocel e, tetring syndrome n=13	5	-	8	-	-		**13(9%)** / **0**
Total	61 (42,4%)	40 (53,3%)	62 (43%)	24 (32%)	21 (14,6%)	11 (14,7%)	**144(100)** / **/75(100%**

Note: Numerator is the main group, denominator is the comparison group,

MC* - Chiari malformation

As shown in the table, in isolated anatomical variants of cystic spinal dysraphism, sensory disturbances were observed in meningoradiculocele in 15 (6.8%), meningomyelocele in 25 (11.4%), myelocystocele in 8 (3.7%), rachisis in 3 (1.4%), Spina bifida complicate in 13 (5.9%) patients.

When meningoradiculocele was combined with other forms of spinal dysplasia with manifestations of spinal cord fixation syndrome (SFCS), sensory disturbances were observed in 54 (68.4%): as meningoradiculocele with tetring - syndrome in 18 (33.3%); meningoradiculocele with tetring syndrome and hydromyelia in 6 (11.1%); meningoradiculocele with hydromyelia and diastematomyelia in 7 (13%); meningoradiculocele with diastematomyelia in 2 (3.7%); meningomyeloradiculocele + syringomyelia in 4 (7.4%); Chiari malformation with meningomyeloradiculocele with tetring syndrome in 8 (14.8%); Chiari malformation, meningomyeloradiculocele with syringomyelia in 9 (16.7%).

In the main group, hypoesthesia was detected in 62 (72.1%) patients and anaesthesia in 21 (65.6%). In the comparison group, hypoesthesia was observed in 24 (31.2%) and anaesthesia in 11 (34.4%) children with loss of sensation in the shins, feet and lower third of the thigh, combined with limitation of movement in the lower extremities.

We assessed the level of cerebral tissue damage using a dermal sensitivity determination scheme according to the spinal cord segments. The upper boundary of the changes was determined by the dominant sensory metamer. In children with severe peripheral paresis, there was a loss or decrease in all types of sensitivity of the conductive type, i.e., downward from the level of cerebral tissue damage. This indicated involvement of the white matter of the spinal cord, its lateral columns with outgoing pathways of pain and temperature sensation; the posterior columns with neurons of musculo-articular, vibration and tactile sensation. By zone of cutaneous innervation, we obtained the following pattern of lesions of different parts of the spinal cord: L1-S3 in 23 (17.6%); L3-S3 in 46 (35.1%) and L5-S3 in 62 (47.3%) of 131 patients with sensory disturbances. In the latter group, there was a predominant reduction or loss of sensitivity in the shins and feet. In the first two groups, 29% (20 patients) of the cases were also noted in the lower third of the thigh.

Analysis of the clinical material showed that out of 87 patients with spinal dysraphism with vegetative and trophic disorders, shortening of the length and circumference of the lower limbs, phenomena of hypotrophy or atrophy of one or both limbs, 69 (79.3%) had hypoesthesia as a sensory disorder. At formation of trophic ulcers in all patients a decrease of sensitivity in the area and around the lesion was noted. Sensory disturbances are very rare in isolation, usually combined with other neurological disorders with more distinct signs in severe and concomitant forms of myelodysplasia.

Chapter summary. Spina bifida aperta is represented by three groups of nosological forms of spinal dysraphism: spina bifida cystica, spina bifida complicate, and Chiari malformation, for which the presence of spinal hernias of different localization and anatomical shape with predominance of envelopocerebral is common. The pathology is predominantly localised in the lumbar region in 76 (34.7%), lumbosacral in 92 (42%), and sacral in 37 (16.9%). In the natural course of this type of spinal dysraphism, patients have bulges of various shapes and sizes with features of the hernial bulge content and its cover. The reason for hospitalization of patients in neonatal and early thoracic age in spina bifida aperta are complications related to the hernial cover. The features of spina bifida complicate are lipomatous and teratoid organoid masses consisting of fragments of individual body parts or miniature structures of individual organs within the herniated protrusion associated with the membranes or substance of the spinal cord.

The clinical manifestations of cystic forms of spinal dysraphism are variable and depend on the localisation, size and anatomical variant. The main clinical manifestations were motor disturbances (88.1%), pelvic dysfunction (76.7%), sensory disturbances (53.9%), trophic disturbances (39.7%), cutaneous stigmas of dysembryogenesis (4.6%) in various combinations. Symptoms of cranial nerve damage in (22.4%) patients were attributed to concomitant hydrocephalus and the consequences of perinatal damage. In MC, general cerebral phenomena were associated with circulatory disturbances in the vertebrobasilar basin and cerebrospinal circulation mainly in the craniovertebral region. The results of comprehensive studies showed a heterogeneous structure of the herniated bulge and the bony component of the hernia. Presented cystic forms of myelodysplasia were found in 140 (63.9%) observations in isolated form, in 79 (36.1%) - in combination with latent forms of spinal dysplasia, aggravating the course, immediate and long-term results of treatment.

In spina bifida aperta, motor disturbances were observed in 88.1% of cases. On the MRS scale, they corresponded to a score of 4 in 9.3%; 3 in 61.7%; 1- 2 in 9.3%; and 0 in 19.7% of children. Impairments were pronounced in severe isolated forms of SMH (48.7%), in combination of SMH with other spinal cord anomalies (40.9%); in spina bifida complicate (10.4%). From 193 patients 87 (45%) had motor disorders accompanied by: trophic disorders in 30 (34.5%); trophic disorders and joint deformities in 35 (40.2%); joint deformities and trophic ulcers in 22 (25.3%). This is explained by the fact that severe and combined variants of osteonerval anomaly have increased spinal malformations with increasing frequency, variants of their combination with the severity of disorders. The frequent combination of locomotor, trophic disorders with deformity in the joints of the lower limb indicates the common pathogenetic mechanisms aggravated by associated vertebro-spinal anomalies, which require early therapeutic and preventive measures to improve the quality of life of patients.

Trophic disorders of the lower extremities were detected in 45.1% of 193 patients with CMH and movement disorders. In 30 (34.5%) patients with trophic disorders, objective examination showed cooling and dry skin with deformation of some toes, thickening of nail plates on the affected side compared to proximal areas and the opposite limb, which was considered to be early vegetotrophic manifestations. In 18 (20,7%) from 87 patients with trophic disturbances, marked chromata, an obvious shortening of length and circumference of the lower limbs in the form of hypotrophy or atrophy with vegetative trophic manifestations of asymmetrical character: on both sides - in 12 (66, 7%), on one side - in 6 (33, 3%) patients.

In 57 (26%) patients with movement disorders, various paralytic deforming arthroses in the joints of the lower limbs, predominantly in the distal direction, were observed. Movement disorders due to subluxation or dislocation of the hip were observed in 24 (42.1%) patients. Six (10.5%) children were wheelchair-bound due to a lack or weakness of the hip extensor and abductor muscles. 18 (31.6%) patients with severe peripheral paresis were able to stand with knee joints supported by the upper extremities. 33 (57.9%) children with various foot deformities walked limp on their own. With severe and extended variants of osteonerval anomaly involving the thoracolumbar spine, 8 (3.6%) out of 219 patients were bedridden, with disproportion in various parts of the body. The data presented indicate that, depending on the level and severity of the neurosegmental lesion, as a result of disproportionate muscle traction and an imbalance of forces between muscle groups of antagonists and synergists, statico-dynamic disturbances contribute to the formation of musculoskeletal pathology in the form of deformities in the joints.

Vegeto-trophic disorders of the lower extremities in spina bifida aperta were detected in 87 (45.1%) of 193 patients with SMH and movement disorders. In 18 (20.7%) of them there was a pronounced shortening of the length and circumference of the lower extremities in the form of hypotrophy or atrophy. At severe forms of spinal pathology in 22 (11.4%) cases trophic disorders were transformed into ulcers of various size and depth with predominant localization in the distal parts of the lower limbs.

Out of 321 patients with neurospinal dysraphism, pelvic organ dysfunction was detected in 270 (84.1%). Pelvic organ dysfunction occurs in both cystic variants 168 (62.2%) and in latent spinal dysraphism 102 (37.8%). The main manifestations of pelvic organ dysfunction are constipation, fecal incontinence, and urinary dysfunction alone or in combination, with varying degrees of severity. For a complete evaluation of the somatic state, neurological status, the dynamics of functional changes in the organs concerned and the establishment of a final diagnosis, consultations with specialists are necessary: a neurologist, a neurosurgeon, a paediatrician and a surgeon.

Urinary dysfunction was manifested as hyperreflexive type in 39 (46.4%) patients of the main group, hyporeflexive type in 19 (22.6%), detrusor-sphincter dyssynergy in 26 (31%) patients. Isolated violation of the defecation act was detected in 63 (29%) patients of the main group out of 217 patients with pelvic disorders. The defecation disorder was observed in the form of chronic constipation in 27 (42.8%) patients; in 28 of them it was combined with urinary disorders. Constipation combined with paradoxical incontinence was observed in 19 (30.2%) patients, in 26 patients it was combined with urinary dysfunction. Anal sphincter insufficiency with faecal incontinence isolated - in 17 (27%) patients (in 16 combined with urinary dysfunction).

Among the neurological manifestations of vertebromedullary anomalies, sensory disturbances are a significant feature, but identifying them causes considerable difficulty in young children. Out of 219 patients with spina bifida aperta, hypoesthesia and anaesthesia were found in 118 (53.9%) observations. The severity of hypoesthesia and anaesthesia of the lower extremities (more often the sole and posterior surface of the tibia) was symmetrical in most cases. Hypoesthesia and anaesthesia in the anogenital region was noted in 41 (18.7%) patients, indicating the involvement of the spinal cord cone in the pathological process.

Chapter V

HIDDEN SPINAL DYSRAPHISM IN THE STRUCTURE OF VERTEBROMEDULLARY ANOMALIES IN CHILDREN

§ 5.1. The role of occult spinal dysraphism in pelvic organ dysfunction, genesis and course of anorectal, urogenital and coloproctal anomalies in children

Concealed spinal dysraphism (CSD) **is an** association of various forms of incomplete mesenchymal, bony structures and/or spinal cord dysplasia without skin integrity, often with hidden clinical and neurological abnormalities of the musculoskeletal system, pelvic organs and other systems. The pathology is predominantly observed in the bony part of the spinal column in the form of vertebral anomalies, relatively rare - spinal dysplasia or a combination of these in different variants. As a rule, myelodysplasias and occult spinal dysraphisms often result in so-called "malformation due to malformation" and/or functional abnormalities of organs in the area corresponding to the segmental innervation of the spinal cord. Of 321 patients with osteonerval anomalies of the spine and spinal cord, spina bifida occulta was detected in 102 (31.8%): in isolated form, without concomitant malformations, in 8 (7.8%), in association with anorectal in 51 (50.0%); urogenital in 13 (12.8%), and in 30 (29.4%) with colorectal abnormalities.

Anorectal and urogenital abnormalities were represented as flush and fistulous forms of rectal atresia, cloaca, infravesical obstruction, and renal and urinary tract malformations. In all cases, these abnormalities were accompanied by defecation or urinary tract abnormalities of varying severity, either isolated or in combination. Among patients with colon anomalies functional disorders in 14 (46,7%) manifested as persistent chronic constipation which was difficult to be treated conservatively, in 2 (6,7%) - as chronic constipation with paradoxical fecal incontinence. Reasons of these disorders were congenital lengthening of sigmoid colon - dolichosigma - in 7 (23,3%); lengthening of large intestine -

dolichocolon - in 14 (46,7%); lengthening and extension of whole colon - megadolichocolon - in 4 (13,3%) or extension of rectum - megarectum - in 5 (16,7%).

The inclusion of this category of patients in the group of latent spinal dysraphism can be explained by the fact that in recent years there has been a marked increase in the number of such patients admitted to the paediatric surgical clinic. At complex examination in them motility disorders of large intestine and functional disorders in the postoperative period from pelvic organs with normal or satisfactory anatomical structure were revealed. In some patients there was no postoperative treatment at all or there was a low, unstable positive effect. At clinical examination of these children various anatomical and functional conditions were revealed: normal anatomical structure and functional condition of anorectal zone - in 41 (40,2%); at normal 39 (38,2%) and satisfactory 14 (13,7%) anatomical structure functional disorders of anorectal zone were revealed in 53 (52,0%); at disturbances of anatomical structure, functional disturbances of anorectal zone - in 8 (7,8%). The presented data indicate that depending on the severity, nature and extent of latent spinal dysraphism, functional disorders are observed in the zone of segmental innervation, with abnormalities in the development of the corresponding organs and systems. This can be explained by the common embryogenesis of these pathologies and anomalies of the distal spine, which confirms the need for targeted examination of each patient for spinal and spinal cord pathology in order to determine the appropriate treatment together with neurologists.

§ 5.2. Clinical and neurological manifestations and paraclinical findings of occult spinal dysraphism with associated anomalies in children

On objective examination in 102 (31.8%) patients with latent spinal dysraphism, one or more cutaneous signs were observed in the zone of split vertebral arches: skin retraction and atrophy or tissue swelling, scarring, pigmentation, coccygeal traction, hemangioma lipomas, hypertrichosis - cutaneous stigmas of disembryogenesis located along the spine or in the perineum. Scoliosis was clearly identified in 10 patients (Table 5.1; Figure 5.1).

Table 5.1

Cutaneous stigmas of dysembryogenesis in patients with occult spinal cord dysraphism (n=102)

Type of stigma	For anorectal anomalies, n=51		For urogenital anomalies, n=13		In abnormalities of the colon, n=30		In isolated spina bifida oculta, n=8	
	abs.	%	abs.	%	abs.	%	abs.	%
Subcutaneous lipoma	2	13,3	0	0	0	0	0	0
Hypertrichosis	1	6,7	0	0	0	0	0	0
Pigmented Nevus	1	6,7	0	0	0	0	0	0
Asymmetry in the folds	4	26,7	2	50,0	2	40,0	0	0
Dermal sinus	0	0,0	1	25,0	1	20,0	0	0
Hemangioma	1	6,7	0	0	0	0	0	0
Scoliosis	6	40,0	1	25,0	2	40,0	0	0
Total	15	62,5	4	16,7	5	20,8	0	0

As shown in Table 5.1, cutaneous stigmata are frequently and variably observed in anorectal and urogenital anomalies. The findings correlate with the number and nature of co-morbid anomalies in these groups. Among patients with ano- and urogenital anomalies there were malformations of various forms with more severe persistent functional disturbances than in patients with elongations of various parts of the colon accompanied by chronic colostasis.

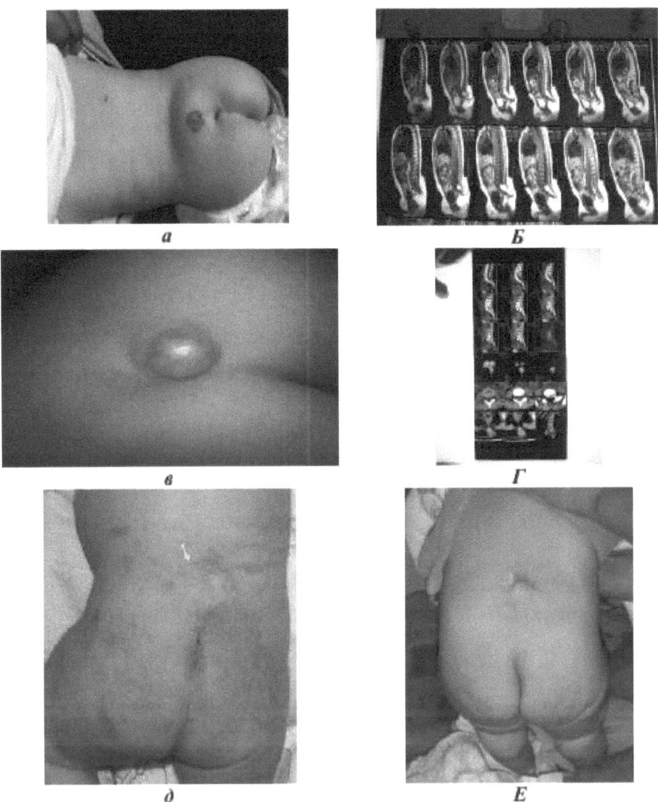

Fig. 5.1. Stigmas of dysembryogenesis in SSD: (a) dermal sinus with hemangioma, patient N. (age 7 months, case no. 234), (b) MRI of the same child - complete cleavage of sacral vertebrae; (c) small cyst (1.0×1.0 cm), patient S. (age 5 months, Blvd. 678/98), d) CT scan of the same child - cleft sacral vertebrae, e) epithelial coccygeal passage with lipomatosis in the lumbar region, patient W.N. (age 4 months, Blvd. 567), f) moderate skin extension in the lumbar region, asymmetry of the buttocks, patient. N.S. (age 7 months, case report no. 6745/78)

Osteoneural anomalies were observed in 94 (92.2%) patients regardless of the severity and form of concomitant anomalies. Our observations indicate that irrespective of the anatomical form of the anorectal and urogenital anomalies, their high association with spinal pathology is observed in the lumbosacral region. Functional and neurological disorders indicate the involvement of spinal struc-

109

tures in the zone of segmental innervation. Among these patients, 15 (14.7%) with severe forms of spinal malformation in 7 (46.7%) and multiple spinal malformations in 8 (53.3%), complex anorectal anomalies such as cloaca, rectovaginal fistulas, rectal sac, vaginal doublings, rectourethral fistulae and urinary system pathology in which even surgical correction does not always provide the desired effect were found. The data presented point to the need for early detection of osteonervous pathology of the spine and spinal cord, regardless of the form of concomitant pathology, and for therapeutic and prophylactic measures.

The type of SSD was verified taking into account the data of functional and instrumental studies: ultrasound, MSCT, MRI of the brain, spinal cord, spinal column; electroneuromyography (ENMG) of the muscles of the lower extremities. Ultrasonography, irrigography, intravenous urography on digital X-ray unit or MSCT were performed to assess anatomical and functional condition of colon and urogenital system. The condition of the vertebrae, the structure and location of the spinal cord cone, and the terminal filament were evaluated. Abnormal development of the spine in the form of lumbosacral dysraphism on the background of rare variants of spinal malformation predominated in this group of patients (Table 5.2).

As shown in Table 5.2, anorectal, urogenital anomalies in 64 (68%) and colorectal anomalies in 30 (32%) patients had SSD as associated anomalies with a predominance of sacroiliac dysraphism (CPD) of 99 (93.4%) (Figure 5.1) over neurospinal (NSD) of 7 (6.6%) (Table 5.2).

Table 5.2

Combined latent spinal dysraphism with anorectal,
urogenital and coloproctal anomalies in children (n=102)

Type of occult spinal dysraphism	For anorectal anomalies n= 51		In urogenital anomalies n=13		For colorectal anomalies n=30		SSD without concomitant anomalies n= 8	
	abs.	%	abs.	%	abs.	%	abs.	%
Posture disorders (sco-	6	10,9	1	7,7	2	6,7	0	0

110

liosis, kyphosis, lordosis)								
Non-retraction of the wishbones:								
- one vertebra	6	10,9	3	23,1	0	0	0	0
- two	12	21,8	3	23,1	8	26,7	6	75,0
- over two	7	12,7	2	15,4	14	46,7	2	25,0
Vertebral body anomaly	2	3,6	2	15 ,4	1	3,3	0	0
Abnormal development of the sacrum (agenesis, dysgenesis, deviation)	4	7,3	1	7,7	2	6,7	0	0
Coccyx anomalies	6	10,9	1	7,7	0	0	0	0
A combination of individual forms	6	10,9	0	0	2	6,7	0	0
Spinal lipomas	2	3,6	0	0	0	0,0	0	0
Tetring syndrome	4	7,3	0	0	1	3,3	0	0
Total	55	51,9	13	12,3	30	28,5	8	7,5

In terms of the nature and frequency of the lesions, the established disorders were more pronounced in anorectal and urogenital anomalies than in colorectal pathology. The difference of causative factors in the genesis of functional disturbances causes a radical difference in intensity and character of neurological disorders. This is confirmed by the presence of somatic, neurological and autonomic disorders in anorectal and urogenital anomalies and the predominance of autonomic disorders with moderate or no somatic, neurological symptomatology in patients with colorectal anomalies.

The incidence of occult spinal dysraphism varied according to the results of comprehensive studies and the nature of the abnormalities detected. Out of 64 patients with anorectal and urogenital abnormalities, 7 (10.9%) had scoliosis as the result of radial methods.

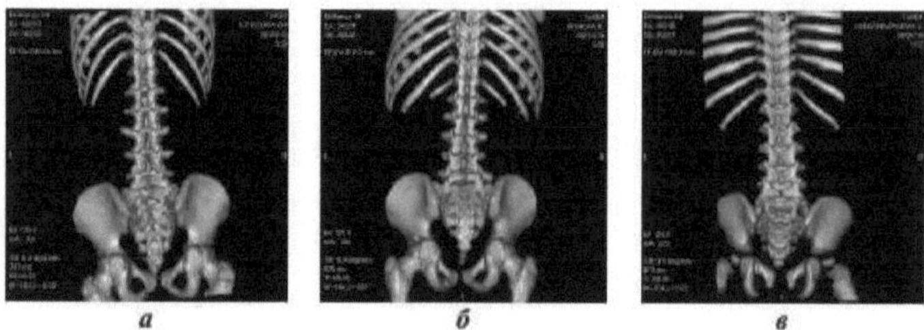

Figure 5.2. Lumbar (a), sacral (a), sacral (b) and sacral (c) arches. (b) and lumbosacral, (c) total split, tethering - coccyx posterior arch syndrome

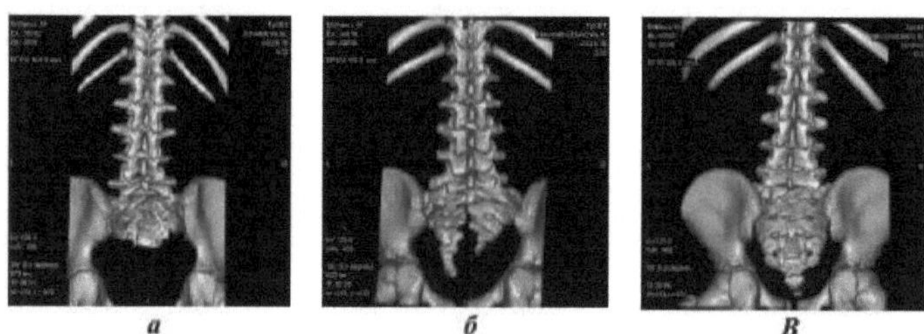

Figure 5.3. Abnormal development of the sacrum: hemisacrum (a), fusion of the sacrum and agenesis of the coccyx (b), semicircumference with agenesis (c)

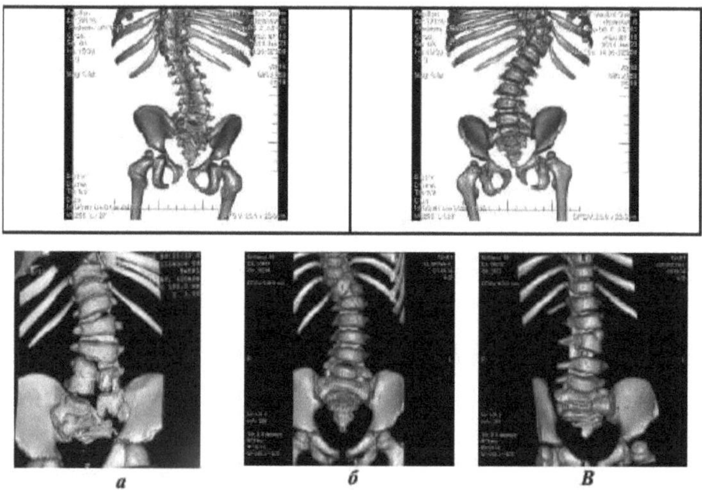

Figure 5.4. Scoliosis: (a) curvature due to the presence of a wedge-shaped vertebrae in the thoracic; b) thoracolumbar; c) lumbar

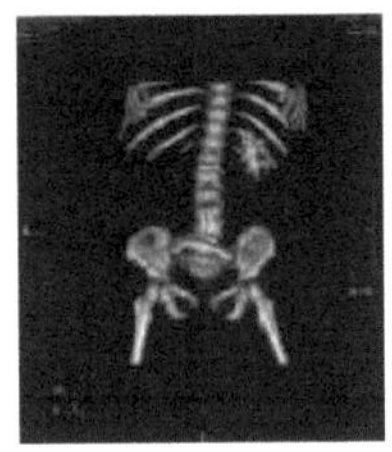 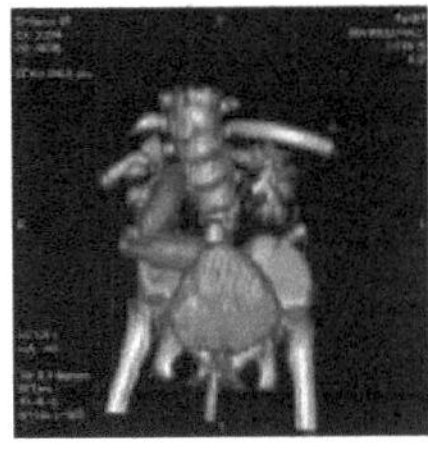 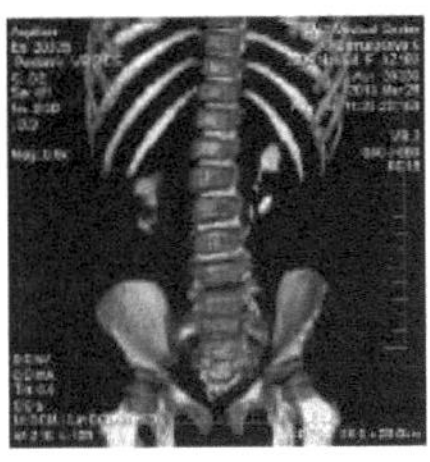

a   б   в

Figure 5.5. Agnesia of the right kidney (a), right-sided ureterohydronephrosis (b); doubling of the left kidney (c).

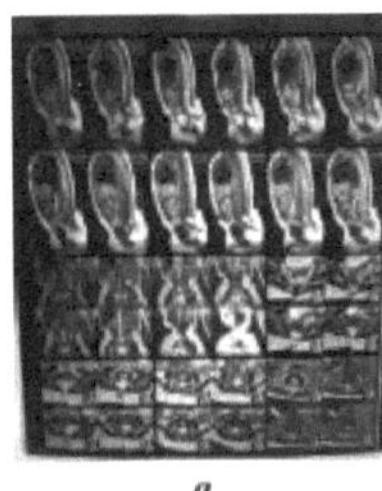 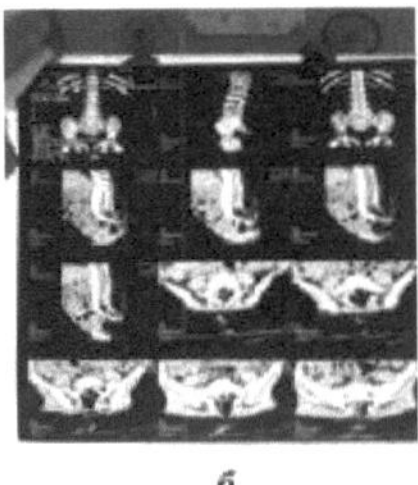 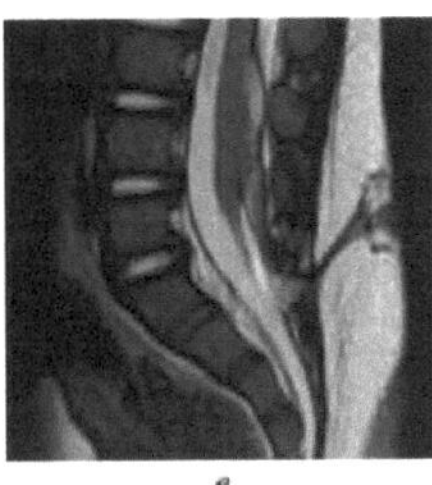

a   б   в

Fig.5.6.Variants of latent spinal dysplasia in latent spinal dysraphism: a) tethering syndrome in urogenital anomaly, patient V.N. (age 2 years, hist. ill. No.566,) b) intradural lipoma, in anorectal anomaly, patient A. D. (age 3 years; case no. 567).

Anomalies of the sacrum and coccyx were found in 12 (54.5%) children. Hypoplasia and agenesis of the coccyx was found in 7 of them, and anomalies of the sacrum in 5. In 33 (51.6%) patients, incompleteness of the vertebral arches was diagnosed predominantly in lumbosacral localization, involving one (9), two or more vertebrae (24). In 6 (6.25%) children, a combination of separate forms of spinal anomalies in the form of nondenaturation and agenesis in different parts was observed. Terminal filament localization in the spinal cord structure was detected on MSCT in 6 cases. In 4 (6.25%) patients, a tetring syndrome was detected, and 2 (3.13%) patients had intradural lipoma.

Out of 30 children with coloproctological anomalies, postural abnormalities were detected in 2 (6.7%), anomalies of sacral development in 2 (6.7%), and anomalies of vertebral bodies with localization in the lumbosacral region in 1. Non-expansion of the vertebral arches in the lumbosacral spine involving two

113

(8) or more vertebrae (14) was diagnosed in 22 (73.3%) patients. Tethering syndrome was diagnosed in 1 (3.3%) patient.

Spina bifida occulta in isolation, detected in 8 patients, was the most common type of occult spinal dysraphism. Non-translocation of the arches of a single vertebra (predominantly lumbar) was observed in only 1 (12.5%) case. In 7 (87.5%) patients, the failure of the arches was observed along two or more vertebrae: localization to the lumbar spine in 2 patients, to the sacral spine in 3 patients, and simultaneous localization to the same extent in 2 patients.

In malformations of the sacrospinous spine, the sacral plexus, whose branches innervate the sphincter apparatus of the bladder and rectum, is affected, which can cause decreased tactile sensitivity of the perineum and functional disorders of various dynamics. Pelvic organ dysfunctions alone or in combination (persistent constipation - 22, chronic constipation with paradoxical fecal incontinence - 14, fecal incontinence - 16; incontinence of feces and urine - 30, incontinence of urine - 20) without marked anorectal anatomical disturbances and predominance of extended flank incompetence in the lumbosacral region covering the areas of interest - S I and SII, does not rule out a role of neurospinal and lumbosacral dysraphism in the genesis of these disorders. Irrespective of the form of concomitant anomaly, the nature and extent of the anorectal dysfunction determines the type and severity of the SSD. In severe dysraphism, the nature of the dysfunction differs in severity. Orthopaedic dysfunction in SSD in the form of hip dysplasia was found in 6 patients and asymmetry of the gluteal folds in 8 patients.

In 13 (12.7%) patients with urinary tract abnormalities we additionally performed MSCT with excretory urography, which provided information on the anatomical and functional state of the kidneys and the urinary system. Agenesis of the right kidney was diagnosed in 3 patients, ureterohydronephrosis - in 8 patients (1 patient had it on both sides); 2 patients had incomplete doubling (1 patient had ectopy of the right ureter in the perineum).

MSCT and contrast-enhanced irrigography performed in 30 (29.4%) patients with colonic pathology made it possible to assess the condition of the colon. In patients with functional disorders of the defecation act, latent spinal dysraphism was represented by less pronounced and rare concomitant forms.

The nature of neurological disorders in SSD depends on the type and severity of vertebral or spinal abnormalities for which the patient was treated (Table 5.3). Of 102 patients, 58 (56.9%) had no detectable neurological abnormalities in the motor or sensory areas. In 44 (43.1%) patients, motor disturbances in the form of paresis (3-4 MRS scores), muscle hypotonia, weakness of the muscles of the lower extremities, and decreased knee reflexes were detected.

Table 5.3

Nature and frequency of neurological manifestations in occult spinal dysraphism combined with ano-rectal, urogenital, coloproctological anomalies (n=102)

Type of neurological disorder	In SSD without concomitant anomalies, n= 8		For anorectal anomalies, n=51		For urogenital anomalies, n=13		For colorectal anomalies, n=30	
	abs	%	abs	%	abs	%	abs	%
Motor disorders	0	0	30	30,9	4	11,8	10	20,8
Sensitivity disorders	0	0	8	8,2	3	8,8	2	4,2
Vegetative violations	0	0	8	8,2	6	17,6	6	12,5
Combined pelvic organ dysfunction	4	50,0	10	10,3	3	8,8	13	27,1
Violations of the act defecation	0	0	36	37,1	0	0,0	16	33,3
Violations of the act urinary incontinence	4	50,0	5	5,2	10	29,4	1	2,1
Abnormal development of other organs	0	0	0	0	8	23,5	0	0
Total	8	4,3	97	51,9	34	18,2	48	25,7

Motor disorders in the form of muscle hypotonia were found in 28 (63.6%) patients, reduced muscle strength and latent paresis in the lower extremities in 9 (20.5%) patients. The examination of 7 (15.9%) patients revealed more pro-

115

nounced neurological symptoms, a combination of motor disorders with foot deformity and disorders of sensory and pelvic organ function. According to the results of complex examinations in these patients, along with the main anomalies of urogenital and anorectal system, more severe forms or a combination of osteonephalous anomalies relating to occult spinal dysraphism were revealed: tetring syndrome was diagnosed in 5 (71.4%) and spinal lipomas in 2 (28.6%) patients. The evaluation of the anal reflex in 29 (28.4%) patients showed weakness of the sphincter apparatus of the rectum.

Sensory disturbances in 13 (12.7%) children were manifested by segmental and radicular changes in the lower limbs and perineum in the form of hypoesthesia. In 7 (53.8%) patients, hypoesthesia was detected in the dermatome that was innervated by roots arising from the level of the split vertebral arches. They were combined with focal neurological disorders in the form of limitation of active movements, muscle hypotonia, vegetotrophic skin and nail disorders, and pelvic organ dysfunction. Examination by radiological diagnostic methods reveals complex combinations of occult spinal dysraphism or extended areas of spinal cleavage. Our observations show that the severity of the sensory disturbances depends on the nature of myelodysplasia and occult spinal dysraphism.

One of the most frequent and unfavourable manifestations of SBS is pelvic dysfunction, which was found in all patients with spina bifida occulta as defecation, urination or a combination of both. Most children showed constipation, intermittent stool puncture, and signs of neurogenic bladder dysfunction in the form of urinary retention or incontinence.

Chapter summary. The early diagnosis of CSD depends above all on the alertness of paediatricians and physicians in other specialties to this pathology. Cutaneous stigmata in the lumbosacral region, the appearance and progression of neurological symptoms with predominant pelvic organ dysfunction in anorectal, urogenital or colorectal abnormalities are evidence of common pathogenetic mechanisms. These findings support the need for targeted screening for hidden spinal, anorectal and urogenital abnormalities.

Our observations indicate that variants of SSD, differing in the nature and extent of cleavage, are often observed in the lumbosacral spine, predominantly on the bone-component side of the spinal column in the form of vertebral anomalies and relatively rarely in spinal dysplasia or a combination thereof. The SSDs, irrespective of the type of nosological forms (vertebral or spinal), proceeded with latent clinical and neurological abnormalities of the pelvic organs. With increasing compression of the dural sac through the bone defect, fixation of spinal roots or spinal cord sections, an increase in neurological symptoms was observed.

Functional and neurological disorders indicate the involvement of spinal structures in the zone of segmental innervation and cause the development of somatic innervation disorders of organs with possible anomalies in the development of relevant organs and systems. Patients with severe forms of myelodysplasia and complex combinations of vertebral anomalies are found to have difficult to correct variants of concomitant malformations with decompensated disorders of their function. The results of the study showed that high combinations of SSD with urogenital, anorectal anomalies or colorectal pathology aggravate their course, adversely affect the results of surgery, and require targeted treatment of functional and residual abnormalities.

The data presented confirm the need for early detection of spinal and spinal cord pathology, regardless of the form of concomitant pathology, and for therapeutic and prophylactic measures.

MRI and MSCT are the main diagnostic modalities for occult spinal dysraphism. When making the final diagnosis, it is important to consider the results of electrophysiological and ultrasound examinations aimed at detecting subclinical neurological abnormalities and the structural and functional states of the organs involved. SSD, regardless of the type of nosological form (vertebral abnormalities or spinal dysplasia), can cause spinal cord fixation syndrome before surgery or at different times after surgery.

Chapter VI

OPTIMISING COMPREHENSIVE TREATMENT AT
SPINAL DYSRAPHISM IN CHILDREN

§ 6.1. Factors influencing the dynamics, course and treatment outcome of spinal dysraphism in children

Surgical treatment for many forms of myelodysplasia is a major component of comprehensive treatment. Of 321 patients with spinal dysraphism, 219 (68.2%) required surgical treatment for cystic forms of spinal dysraphism. Surgical interventions were performed in 198 (90.4%) patients. In 21 (9.6%) patients (12 in the main group, 9 in comparison group) not operated due to inoperability (multiple malformations incompatible with life, socially unadaptable complications with parental consent to refusal) surgical intervention was not performed In 21 (9.6%) cases with severe forms of SMH (rachyschisis - 3, giant myelocystocele - 4, myelomeningocele - 4, and in combination of severe forms of SMH with complex malformations of other organs and systems, accompanied by severe complications of spinal pathology and combined anomalies - 6 patients were not operated upon by collegial decision of medical personnel of different specialities with the consent of parents of the child - accepting the process as incurable. 4 patients did not undergo surgical treatment due to parental refusal. Surgical treatment in 20 (10.1%) patients was performed at the age of 1-28 days because of emergency indications (in case of ruptured membranes - 3-15%, in case of acute thinning of membranes with menace of liquorrhea - 11-55%, in 6 (30%) patients - due to the progressing pyoinflammatory changes in membranes with increasing meningoencephalitis phenomena). In 103 (52,02%) patients surgical intervention was performed routinely at the age of 1 month to 1 year. 69 (34,85%) children were operated at the age of 1-12 years. 6 (3.03%) children were operated on at the age of 12-16 years.

Osteonephalic anomalies are congenital abnormalities, as other malformations in isolation are rare, multiple lesions are often observed, and the variant "malformation due to malformation" is not excluded. In patients with cystic spinal dysraphism 89 (40.6%) had combined malformations of other organs and systems: cardiovascular system - 7 (7.9%); musculoskeletal system (scoliosis, kyphosis) - 19 (21.3%); gastrointestinal tract - 4 (4.5%); urogenital system - 4 (4.5%); multiple malformations of 1 (1.1%). This group of patients had functional disorders in the area of segmental innervation of spinal cord lesion: dysfunction of pelvic organs - 168 (76.7%); orthopedic problems - 57 (26%); trophic disorders - 87 (39.7%), which required special investigation methods and appropriate treatment courses.

102 patients with latent spinal dysraphism with concomitant developmental anomalies who underwent surgeries in the profile of the established pathology underwent special methods of investigation providing for revealing the character of the main pathology (anorectal, urogenital, coloproctological) and concomitant latent spinal dysraphism. In 94 (92%) patients the nature of spinal dysraphism was established at the stage of follow-up. They underwent surgery not for spinal pathology, but for correction of underlying pathology associated with anorectal, urogenital or colorectal abnormalities. In the course of a comprehensive examination, 98 anomalies relating to occult spinal dysraphism were identified. Patients were in need of conservative medicament and physiotherapeutic treatment courses for correction of existent functional disturbances caused or aggravated by hidden spinal dysraphism. The presented data indicate that cystic and latent forms of spinal dysraphism are characterized by a high combination of functional disorders or with anomalies of the anorectal, urogenital and gastrointestinal organs innervated by branches of the most frequently affected spinal cord zone - lumbosacral region.

There is no doubt that surgical treatment of a spinal hernia is not only a cosmetic repair of the hernia, but should also be aimed at correcting concomitant anomalies, the resulting secondary anthomo-functional disorders on the part of other organs and systems, with systematic courses of rehabilitation treatment. The analysis of medical documents of the patients from the comparison group and patients, who received treatment (primary, repeated) in other various departments (neurosurgery, surgery, neurology) showed, that the therapeutic-diagnostic tactics was chosen in accordance with the profile of the establishment. We studied the anamnestic data of 10 (5%) out of 198 operated patients with SMG who were admitted from other medical institutions and underwent surgical treatment consisting only of excision of the hernia without the appropriate treatment of secondary changes. On discharge from hospital, the parents of the patients were not advised of the need for treatment by appropriate specialists. As a result, urinary and/or defecation disorders were predominant due to the progression of residual phenomena. The patients were repeatedly referred to various clinics.

In the surgical wards, spinal dysraphism was given little or no attention when concomitant pathology (anorectal, urogenital) was sufficiently identified. In the pathology of the identified abnormalities, accordingly, in the vast majority of cases, patients had persistent functional impairments, some of them with a tendency to progress.

The type of pelvic organ dysfunction was not taken into account in the treatment of defecation or urination disorders in the neurology departments. The lack of a systematic approach and continuity between specialists in the organization of comprehensive treatment of patients with spinal malformations seems to be one of the main reasons for the high disappointing treatment results.

In the genesis of the progression of neurological symptoms and residual phenomena can be attributed in no small measure to the neglect of special research methods, among patients in the comparison group - 12 (16%) and 6 (4.2%) patients in the main group underwent emergency surgery in neonatal and early breast age due to the complications (ruptured membranes, pyoinflammatory complications) of cystic forms of spinal dysraphism without performing CT and MRI studies. As a result, in some of these patients, combined forms of spinal dysplasia (syringomyelia, tetring syndrome, hydromyelia, and/or complex variants of vertebral anomalies) remained undetected, which subsequently caused the development of spinal cord fixation syndrome, with its corresponding manifestations. The dynamics of neurological abnormalities before and after treatment in comparison patients are shown in Table 6.1.

Table 6.1

The nature of the initial neurological abnormalities and their development after

of patients with spinal dysraphism in the comparison group

Types of irregularities detected on initial admission	Number of people examined over time (n=45)		Dynamic results					
			Positive dynamics		Without momentum		Negative dynamics	
	abs.	%	abs	%	abs	%	abs	%
Spina bifida aperta								
- propulsion	34	34,3	11	50,0	18	30,0	5	29,4
- trophic	18	18,2	4	18,2	10	16,7	4	23,5
- sensitive	20	20,2	3	13,6	17	28,3	0	0,0
- Pelvic organ dysfunction	27	27,3	4	18,2	15	25,0	8	47,1
Spina bifida oculta								
(a) Pelvic organ dysfunction (n=2)	2	100,0	1	100,0	1	100,0	0	0

As can be seen from the table, among the observed 77 patients in the comparison group, the dynamics of the neurological status of cystic forms was observed in 45 (58.4%) patients. Sixty-eight (88.3%) children were discharged from the hospital, in 9 (11.6%) patients not included in the dynamic control group the pathology was considered inoperable, 3 of them (33.3%) died within 3-4 months after discharge from the hospital from various complications. In 45 examined patients discharged from the hospital, different dynamics of some neurological manifestations were revealed before and after operation: no appreciable changes were revealed in 18 (52,9%) cases, in 11 (32,4%) a moderate positive dynamic of lower limb movements was registered, in 5 (14,7%) cases negative dynamics was diagnosed. It should be noted that the immediate and long-term results in terms of neurological status depend on the severity of myelodysplasia. When analyzing the data, the best results were observed in uncomplicated forms of osteonephritic anomaly and usually among those operated on early, including in the neonatal period with appropriate indications for urgent or elective surgery. Not all patients in the comparison group underwent systematic rehabilitation. Two patients in this group underwent repeated surgeries for primary or secondary spinal cord fixation in various foreign clinics. However, the results of these operations were also disappointing.

§ 6.2. The importance of a multidisciplinary approach in optimising the comprehensive treatment of spinal dysraphism in children.

Based on the analysis of the above data and taking into account diagnostic and tactical errors made by doctors of various institutions, we used an early multidisciplinary approach with the participation of various specialists in diagnosis and treatment according to the nature of the combined pathology in order to optimize therapeutic and diagnostic tactics in patients with spinal malformations. The basic principles of this approach consist in a comprehensive examination of patients aimed at establishing the nature of spinal and combined pathology and active detection of latent spinal dysraphism and related functional disorders, as well as early prophylactic and therapeutic measures.

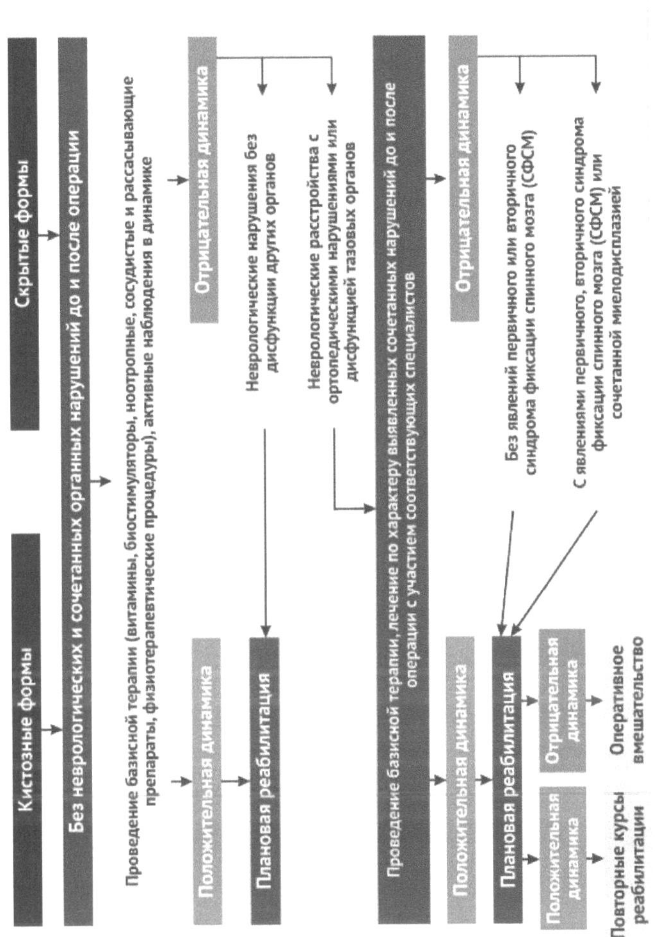

Figure 6.1. Treatment algorithm for spinal dysraphia

Early preventive drug therapy (symptomatic, vascular, nootropic drugs, vitamin therapy and physiotherapeutic procedures (massage, exercise therapy, drug electrophoresis) were included in the treatment package. Targeted treatment from 2-3 weeks after surgery was also carried out in patients in the main group with spinal malformations according to the nature of pelvic organ dysfunction and orthopaedic disorders with the participation of a pediatric surgeon, urologist and orthopaedist.

Patients were treated with a complex baseline treatment with drugs affecting the neurotransmitter systems of the brain. This reduced the severity or progression of central and peripheral disorders. Depending on age and body weight, patients were prescribed neurotransmitters (encephabol, cerebrolysin, cortexin, piracetam, pantocalcin, glutamic acid); vitamins (B, C, A, E); blood circulation improvers (cinnarizine, nicotinic acid, cytochrome); biostimulants, resolving drugs (aloe, lidase). Neurotransmitter amino acids in the beginning were pre-scribed parenterally (Cortexin 5-10 mg, Piracetam 50 mg/kg/day) for 10 days in injections, then in tablets. Pantocalcin 250 mg, glycine 50 mg/kg/day for 30-40 days.

The main principles of treatment used in the main group of patients begin with pelvic organ dysfunction, which is the most common and the most diverse of the neurological disorders observed in patients with spinal dysraphism. Pelvic organ dysfunction in spinal dysraphism occurs early in a child's life and may cause secondary changes in the urinary or digestive tract. The child's quality of life may be impaired when other neurological abnormalities are present. Therefore, early identification of the disorder and targeted treatment can improve the im-mediate and long-term results of comprehensive treatment. There is no universal treatment for pelvic organ dysfunctions in children with spinal disorders. An in-dividual approach should be taken depending on the nature of the disorder. Con-sideration of the type of dysfunction increases the effectiveness of comprehen-sive treatment. Therapy for bladder dysfunction (BFD) is usually aimed at re-ducing the pressure in a hypertensive bladder or at increasing the resistance of the bladder outlet to achieve urine retention. When the bladder is hypotonic, the contractility of the detrusor should be increased. When a hypotonic neurogenic bladder is unable to contract, a complex variant of bladder dysfunction develops under conditions of increased resistance of the bladder outlet, which is difficult to treat. Antibiotics and uroseptics have been prescribed for microbial inflammation of the urinary tract, regardless of the type of urinary dysfunction.

In hyporeflexive detrusor dysfunction in 19 (22.6%) children, in order to reduce bladder capacity, increase its sensitivity to stretching and timely occurrence of urge to urination, it is necessary to accustom the child to the emptying of the bladder at certain times of the day in two steps. This approach is effective for children who can consciously regulate the act of urination, i.e. at an older age. In young children, periodic catheterisation with bladder emptying 2-3 times a day was carried out for this purpose. If bladder atony is pronounced, during the first week a permanent urine diversion through a catheter left in the detrusor cavity was resorted to. During the next 7 days the bladder was emptied every 4 hours by opening the urinary catheter. This tactic helps to reduce the size of the bladder and reduces the volume of accumulated and residual urine. Medication correction involved stimulation of detrusor bladder activity. Nivalin was administered intramuscularly for 10 days, followed by 30-40 days of tablets. In children under one year of age, electrophoresis with nivalin was carried out in the bladder area. Nivalin increases the intensity of the nerve impulse to the muscle tissue, increases muscle contraction and its duration, stimulates detrusor function of the bladder, reduces intravesical pressure by blocking hypertonic contractions. Patients were also treated with sinusoidal modulated currents on the bladder area, physical therapy, and general massage.

In the hyperreflexive type in 39 (46.4%), when the bladder capacity is below age-specific values with a relative increase in intravesical pressure, permanent catheterisation was effective in adapting the organ to the increase in the initial high intravesical pressure against the background of increased hydraulic pressure. A catheter was inserted into the bladder, through which a physiological solution with antibiotics or a 1:5000 solution of furacilin was injected at 50% of the organ's age capacity. The catheter was closed for four hours, then the bladder was emptied completely and the total contents measured. The difference between injected and excreted fluid was used to determine the bladder capacity and the volume of the child's diuresis over four hours. From 8 to 24 hours, the manipulation was repeated every 4 hours, increasing the injected fluid by 10 ml more than the previous one. From 24 to 8 am the catheter was closed. Sessions of dosed increase of intravesical pressure were carried out for 7-10 days. Ultrasonography was used to check bladder size and the occurrence of vesicoureteral reflux daily at the beginning and end of the manipulation. The urethral catheter was changed every 3-4 days. The course of treatment was repeated after three months. Drug therapy for hyperreflexive bladder included m-cholinolytics, atropine by electrophoresis on the bladder area for 5 days; Driptan 2.5-5 mg 2-3 times daily for 1-2 months; sedative therapy before bedtime (biopassitis, novopassit, motherwort) in an age-appropriate dosage.

Drug therapy was combined with physiotherapy (electrophoresis with atropine or eufillin, sinusoidal modulated currents, low-energy laser, application of paraffin or ozokerite to the bladder and lumbosacral area) to inhibit the effects on bladder ganglion and myocytes.

In detrusor-sphincter dyssynergy in 26(31%), local treatment was similar to that for the hyperreflexive type of bladder disorder, as there is a high incidence of detrusor instability in this type. Typically, bladder capacity is lower than age-matched with relatively high intravesical pressure. Continuous catheterisation to adapt the organ to the increasing initial intravesical pressure is therefore of great importance. Drug therapy was combined with physiotherapy (electrophoresis with atropine or eufillin, sinusoidal modulated currents, low-energy laser, application of paraffin or ozokerite to the bladder and lumbosacral area), which have an inhibitory effect on the bladder ganglion and myocytes.

In the treatment of constipation 27 (42.6%), regular emptying of the rectum, nutritional therapy and an individuated diet are of paramount importance. The intake of 4-5 tablespoons (teaspoons for small children) of mineral oils (olive oil, linseed oil, sunflower oil) helps to normalise defecation and the consistency of faeces. Children over 3 years of age are taught to regularly empty their bowels voluntarily every day at the same time for 10-20 minutes. This is best done shortly after a meal to take advantage of the gastrointestinal reflex that occurs after a meal. In the absence of independent stools, purging enemas have been used. Hyporeflexor dysfunction was stimulated by galantamine hydrobromide intramuscularly for 10 days, and subsequently by tablets for 30-40 days. Therapeutic exercises to strengthen the abdominal abs and perineum muscles, tonic massage of the anterior abdominal wall, long back muscles and lumbar region and laser therapy were carried out; dysbacteriosis correction was prescribed.

In defecation disorders with anal sphincter insufficiency 17 (27%), therapeutic measures aimed at training and strengthening the retention apparatus of the rectum in the form of purging and training enemas, gradually increasing the amount of fluid administered and prolonging retention time in the rectum are of particular importance. Electrical stimulation of the sphincter apparatus and mechanical training on a rubber tube were carried out. By inserting the gas tube into the anal canal to a depth of 4-5 cm, the child was taught to squeeze and relax the sphincter not with the gluteal muscles but with the anal compressor. The manipulation was repeated for 2-3 minutes 4 times a day.

In the combined disorder of constipation and paradoxical faecal incontinence, 19 (30.2%) patients were treated with the complex measures used in chronic colostasis and anal sphincter insufficiency.

When defecation disorders were combined with urinary disorders, 70 (32.3%) patients were treated according to the nature of the defecation disorder.

Motor disorders are one of the frequent clinical manifestations of spinal pathology whose presence and severity depend on the type, degree and level of myelodysplasia. These disorders are often accompanied by symmetrical or asymmetrical deformities and abnormalities in the joints of the lower limbs with an increase in their frequency in the distal direction. The most common type of such abnormality is the equinus position of the feet. Muscle traction and force imbalances between antagonist and synergist muscle groups due to innervation disorders are the main cause of musculoskeletal system pathology and static-dynamic disturbances resulting in instability of vertical stability and movements in the lower extremities. Pathological deformities in spinal pathology are less fixed in most young patients. Early repeated courses of massage, physiotherapeutic procedures and casts correction in 12 (21%) out of 57 patients with different deformities and pathologies of lower limb joints (deformity, dislocation, dysplasia) against complex basic therapy provided positive results: in 3 (25%) cases dysplasia phenomena in hip joints were eliminated, in 9 (75%) patients further deformation progression was eliminated or stopped.

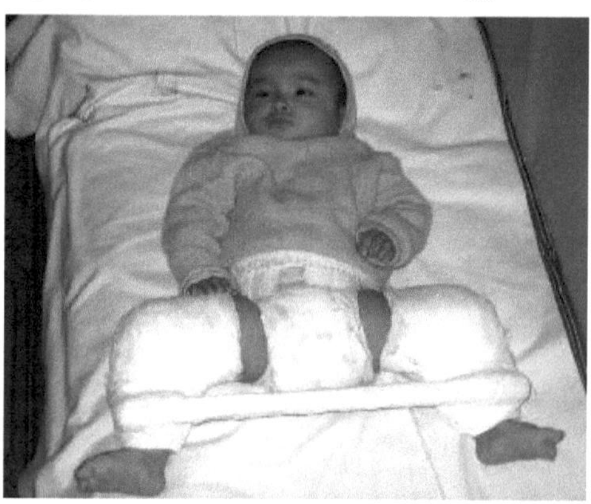

Figure 6.2. Patient A.W., 8 months old. Is.b.no.

These conservative measures also help to prevent the progression of trophic disorders and the formation of trophic ulcers. Systematic measures to reduce spasticity and improve microcirculation in the lower extremities with physiotherapeutic procedures (constant hygiene, massages, local laser irradiation, dressings with heparin ointment) and medication are the basis of basic prevention of trophic disorders.

Treatment of trophic-necrotic lesions (22 patients) was limited to reduction of intoxication, correction of anemia, hypoproteinemia and antibacterial therapy, taking into account the antibiotic profile. The complex of treatment included vitamins (B, C, A, E) immunomodilators (aloe, lidase, fibs) and drugs of rheological and vasodilatory action that improve microcirculation (trental, nicotinic acid). The arsenal of local physiotherapy (UVB, UHF, electrophoresis with novocaine, antibiotics) is widely used. Local conservative treatment consisted in wound cleansing and repeated dressings with preparations, providing wound cleansing, stimulation of regeneration processes (Levomikol ointment, Solcoseryl, Actovegin, Betadin). Fargals, a solution for external application, which has antiseptic, antimicrobial and wound-healing properties, was found to be effective. Complete healing of trophic ulcers occurred in patients with localization of the process in the back and in the proximal parts of the lower limbs. In trophic ulcers of the fingers and plantar surface of the feet there was only clearing of the wound without a tendency to reduce its size. Surgical intervention was performed after sanation of the trophic ulcer surface. At excision of necrotic tissues with plasty by a displaced skin flap, in three of 5 patients we managed to achieve partial edge convergence, in two patients sutures diverged. Therefore, we prefer to apply delayed sutures after the cleansing and emergence of granulation tissue, which usually occurs on the 10th-12th day after manipulation.

In the case of trophic osteomyelitis (2 patients), sanation and removal of destructive areas of the affected bone were carried out, hemostasis was achieved using electrocoagulation, the wound was filled with antibiotics and sutures were placed to close the wound edges with the insertion of a rubber outlet. The tibia and foot were fixed in the initial position of the ankle joint with a removable plaster cast for daily dressings. In the postoperative period the complex of treatment included infra-red pulse laser therapy with the device "Vostok" (Russia) with the parameters of radiation power density up to (100mVt/cm2) in the course of 5 minutes, 5-7 sessions. Relapse or exacerbation of the process was observed in 1 patient.

The effectiveness of the multidisciplinary approach is also confirmed by the positive results of the treatment of 102 patients with spina bifida occulta who underwent surgery for associated anomalies (anorectal, urogenital, colon anomalies) and appropriate courses of conservative therapy for functional disorders caused by occult spinal dysraphism.

The effectiveness of our proposed tactics for cystic and occult forms of spinal dysraphism is evidenced by the dynamics of basic neurological disorders in 232 (95%) of the 244 patients observed in the main group (Table 6.2).

Table 6.2

The nature of the initial neurological abnormalities and their development after
The following are the results of the treatment of patients in the main group with spinal dysraphism (n=232)

Type and total number of abnormalities detected on initial admission Spina bifida aperta (n=144)	Number of people surveyed over time (n=232)		Dynamic results					
			Positive dynamics		Without momentum		Negative dynamics	
	abs.	%	abs	%	abs	%	abs	%
Spina bifida aperta (n=144)								
- motor (n=132)	132	33,8	29	35,4	91	34,1	12	28,6
- trophic (n=59)	59	15,1	6	7,3	43	16,1	10	23,8
- sensitive(n=83)	83	21,2	12	14,6	63	23,6	8	19,0*
- Pelvic organ dysfunction (n=117)	117	29,9	35	42,7*	70	26,2	12	28,6
Spina bifida okulta (n=100)								
(a) Motor (n=44)	44	19	10	26,3	31	28,4	3	30,0
c) sensitive(n=13)	13	5,6	3	7,9	10	9,2	0	0
d) Pelvic organ dysfunction (n=100)	100	43,1***	25	65,8***	68	62,4***	7	30,0

Note: * - differences from comparison group (see Table 6.1) are significant (* - P<0.05, *** - P<0.001)

As can be seen from this table, the dynamics of neurological disorders during the treatment stages of spinal pathology can manifest themselves in different ways: remaining unchanged, with positive or negative results. Among the disorders, trophic disorders tend to be progressive, while sensory disorders are more stable. A clear positive dynamics was observed in the motor sphere and pelvic organ dysfunction in patients with systematic repeated courses of supportive therapy. Therefore, the patients were under outpatient monitoring with repeated

130

10-15 day courses of treatment in an outpatient clinic or hospital every 3-4 months for 2 years, and later - twice a year.

Thus, out of 77 patients in the comparison group 68 (88,3%) children were discharged from the hospital, a lethal outcome was observed in 3 (3,9%) cases. In the study group 232 (95%) out of 244 patients were discharged, lethal outcome was observed in 4 (1.7%) cases. Long-term results of treatment from 6 months to 4 years were traced in 232 patients of the main group and in 45 (60,8%) patients of the comparison group. To facilitate a comparative analysis of treatment in the study groups, long-term outcomes were assessed according to the following criteria: good, satisfactory, unsatisfactory (Table 6,3).

Table 6.3

A comparative assessment of the long-term outcomes of patients with spinal dysraphism according to the criteria compiled.

Type of spinal Dysraphism	Number Surveyed		Good		Satisfactory		Not satisfactory	
	abs.	%	abs.	%	abs.	%	abs.	%
Spina bifida aperta n=132/43	132	46,9	43	63,2*	72	51,4***	17	12,9**
	43	95,6	9	90,0	23	53,5	11	100,0
Spina bifida okulta n=100/2	100	43,1	25	36,8*	68	48,6***	7	7
	2	4,4	1	10,0	1	50	0	0

Note: in number - main group; in denominator - comparison group, * - differences relative to comparison group data are significant (* - P<0.05, ** - P<0.01, *** - P<0.001)

The result was considered good - 78 (28.2%) in the absence of complaints, neurological symptoms and residual phenomena, the patient was fully socially adapted and was not registered for disability. 164 (59,2%) were considered satisfactory in the presence of positive dynamics, preservation of moderate residual phenomena and no signs of spinal cord fixation syndrome according to MRI findings. The patient is partially socially adapted. He receives a disability allowance. Unsatisfactory result - 35 (12,6%) considered as no positive dynamics or negative dynamics after repeated courses of rehabilitation therapy.

131

Signs of spinal dysplasia or spinal cord fixation syndrome were detected on MRI examinations. Patient is socially maladjusted. Disability since childhood. The data presented indicate that a multidisciplinary approach involving specialists (neurologist, neurosurgeon, orthopaedist, pediatric surgeon, urologist) and dynamic monitoring with appropriate courses of special, medication and physiotherapeutic treatment in patients in the main group contributed to better results and improved quality of life in the main group patients compared to the control group. The optimisation of diagnostics for the identification of the nature of spinal pathology and the active detection of hidden dysraphism are also of great importance.

Chapter summary.

The results of the complex treatment of myelodysplasia largely depend on the status of neurological status depending on the nature and severity of spinal malformations. In the natural course of the pathological process among the unoperated as well as in some of the operated patients, progression of the disease with the intensification of all the clinical signs, with the tendency to develop secondary complications of inflammatory nature and trophic disorders, which confirm the need for early diagnosis and timely implementation of appropriate treatment tactics. Surgical treatment of cystic forms of spinal malformations is the main method of not only cosmetic elimination of herniation, but also should be aimed at maximum radical correction of osteneural anomaly with combined myelodysplasia with measures to prevent fixed spinal cord syndrome and resulting secondary anthomo-functional disorders of the organs and systems involved. Early comprehensive correction of myelodysplasia, orthopedic disorders, urological and coloproctologic dysfunctions prevents their progression and significantly reduces the risk of neurological deficit and improves the quality of life of patients. Children who have undergone surgery need to be dynamically monitored, with examination by related specialists and repeated courses of rehabilitation therapy. The progression of neurological symptoms and residual phenomena in some patients indicates repeated or secondary fixation of various parts of

the spinal cord. In such cases, the management of the patient is complex and
sometimes requires repeated neurosurgical operations.

CONCLUSION

Spinal dysraphism is a diverse group of malformations of the spine and spinal cord and occupies a leading place in the structure of spinal pathology (traumatic, infectious and tumour origin) and malformations of the central nervous system (CNS). Many forms of Spina bifida are compatible with life, with a mortality rate of 10% in complex forms. However, the observed residual phenomena of a functional and organic nature persist even after surgical correction, which has not only medical but also social significance. The majority of works devoted to the diagnosis and treatment of myelodysplasia reflect surgical aspects, consider urodynamic, colodynamic complications of spinal hernia and locomotor disorders separately; but do not contain a comprehensive assessment of the combined polymorphic disorders and do not cover their treatment methods sufficiently.

The aim of this study is to optimise early diagnosis, improve treatment outcomes and, on this basis, improve the quality of life and social adjustment of children with osteonerval anomalies of the spine and spinal cord.

The work was based on the analysis of diagnosis and treatment results of 321 patients (156(48.6%) boys and 165(51.4%) girls) aged from one day to 18 years with spinal dysraphism of various forms in combination with other types of spinal malformations and abnormalities of other organs and systems. The patients were divided into two groups. The comparison group consisted of 77 (24%) patients followed up from 2000 to 2011 and examined using conventional methods. The main group consisted of 244 (76%) patients observed between 2012 and 2016. In this group of patients spinal pathology was verified taking into account the results of functional and instrumental examinations of the spine, spinal cord and internal organs. In 219 (68.2%) patients, variants of spinal dysraphism were observed in different clinical and morphological forms of spinal hernia. Of 102 (31.8%), 51 (50%) patients had occult forms of spinal dysraphism associated with anorectal; 13 (12.75%) had urogenital abnormalities; and 30 (29.41%) had colorectal pathology. In 8 (7.84%) patients spina bifida occulta was diagnosed in isolation with disorders of the act of defecation and urination. The predominance of spinal anomalies in the form of lumbosacral dysraphism on the background of rare variants of spinal malformation is characteristic of this group of patients. Localization of spinal dysraphism along the spinal column varied, regardless of the type (open or occult), the predominant location was in the lumbosacral region.

Verification of ostenevular anomalies in the form of isolated or combined anomalies of the spine and/or spinal cord with overt or covert manifestations of spinal lesions was performed taking into account the clinical and neurological status and results of functional and instrumental studies at admission, at the stages of treatment (at discharge from hospital, 2 and 6 months after discharge, delayed to 1 year and remote within 1-5 years) in inpatient and outpatient conditions. Extremely diverse and polymorphic in their manifestations, they were observed in children of all age groups.

Of 219 (68.2%) patients with cystic spinal hernia (CSH) of predominantly lumbosacral localisation in 135 (61.6%); it was combined with tertoid and lipomatous masses - spina bifida complicate - in 32 (14.6%); Chiari malformation in 26 (11.9%) and rachyschisis in 3 (1.4%).

Hidden cleft - spina bifida oculta - in 102 (31.8%) patients as anomalies of the spine was found in 8 (7.8%) patients in isolated form, in 94 (92.2%) - in combination with other anomalies; impaired pelvic organ function was common for all. In such cases, in addition to nephrourological and proctological examination aimed at detecting anatomical-functional, urodynamic and colodynamic abnormalities, the type of spinal pathology was necessarily determined. Spinal abnormalities of various forms and extent were noted in 62 (60.8%) patients in the lumbosacral region.

The main significance in the diagnosis of spinal malformations is the neurological examination of the patient, aimed at establishing the topography of the spinal cord lesion. Comparing the symptoms of local segmental lesions of the spinal cord with the prevalence of conductive motor and sensory disturbances and the nature of changes in pelvic organ function allows us to accurately establish the localization of the pathological focus, its volume and characteristic local changes. The main clinical diagnosis was based on the clinical manifestations and the results of auxiliary examination methods.

On clinical examination, 148 (46.1%) patients had spinal malformations considered to be an isolated malformation. It should be emphasised that the isolation of the malformation is conditional, as other anomalies may go undetected due to the incomplete examination of patients. Currently, the presence of a spinal hernia or signs of CSD in a patient is considered a marker for potential malformations of the central nervous system and other body systems and necessarily requires an examination aimed at detecting concomitant anomalies of the CNS and other organs and systems.

Examinations with the use of specific methods revealed hidden variants of myelodysplasia in SMH and dysplastic changes of the spine as variants of hidden spinal dysraphism. In 219 (68.2%) cases of spina bifida apperta, 79(39%) additional variants of myelodysplasia were identified, aggravating the course and outcome of the disease. The incidence of these anomalies was unequal in our observations. In the comparison group of 17 children with combined forms of myelodysplasia, 6 (35.2%) underwent no preoperative CT or MRI studies. Due to the progression of neurological symptoms after surgery, repeated examinations in these patients revealed one of the variants of spinal cord fixation syndrome. With the increased use of special methods of investigation in the main group, the detection of combined anomalies of the spinal cord, spine, and other organs and systems has increased.

Among patients with occult forms of spinal dysraphism, spinal anomalies predominated in 83(84.7%) cases compared with myelodysplasia. In the case of unexpressed spinal anomalies (non-dislocation of one vertebral arch, moderate scoliosis, hypoplasia of coccyx), functional disorders of the "concerned" organs in the zone of segmental innervation and autonomic disorders were observed in 31 (30.4%) patients. In more severe osteonerval anomalies, 15 (15.3%) patients had neurological, urogenital, or coloproctological abnormalities in addition to the above mentioned disorders. Spinal malformations are not only characterized by a combination of different osteonephalic anomalies. In 20% of patients, malformations of other organs and systems were observed, mutually aggravating the course of the disease and quality of life. The findings on the prevalence of combined and multiple lesions allow congenital spinal malformations to be classified as multiple malformations.

The diagnosis of spinal malformations consists of antenatal and early postnatal diagnosis. To improve diagnosis, the clinical alertness of allied paediatric professionals should be increased and targeted examinations should be carried out in the following circumstances:

- the birth of a child with spinal malformations established antenatally;

- the presence of clear clinical manifestations of cystic CMH in the child;

- Posture disorders and spinal deformities;

- cutaneous stigma of dysembryogenesis with characteristic localisation along the spinal column;

- urogenital and coloproctological anomalies;

- the presence of asymmetry and trophic phenomena in the lower limb;

- the presence of neurological (motor, sensory) symptoms;

- Dysfunction of urination and defecation in the absence of anatomical abnormalities of the pelvic and perineal organs;

- surgical intervention for spinal dysraphism, after which residual phenomena appear or progress.

Out of 219 (68.2%) patients with spinal dysraphism, splitting of the spine with the formation of a cystic mass in the form of a spinal hernia was detected in 161 (73.5%); spina bifida complicate including different anatomical forms of spinal hernia and dystopic formation of lipoma, fibrous tissue or teratoid inclusions around hernial protrusion - 32 (14.6%); Chiari malformation (MC) of types I and II combined with meningocele or meningomyelocele in 26 (11.9%). These nosological forms are characterized by cerebrospinal hernias of different localization and anatomical form, which differ in their clinical and anatomical features. The determining factor in the course, severity of clinical and neurological symptoms, and prognosis of these forms of spinal dysraphism is the content of the hernial sac. The envelope-brain forms were noted in 192 (87.7%); meningocele in 24 (11%); complete cleavage in 3 (1.3%) patients. The localization, size, and shape of the hernial protrusion also determine the severity of clinical and neurological symptoms, since the area of the defect along the spinal column and the zone of segmental innervation vary. The condition of the herniated cover affects the occurrence of complications of a purulent and inflammatory nature, which may subsequently cause the development of spinal cord fixation syndrome.

A special feature of Spina bifida complicate is the presence of lipomatous and teratoid masses often of an organoid nature consisting of fragments of individual body parts or presented as a miniature structure of individual organs within the herniated bulge associated with the membrane or substance of the spinal cord.

The clinical manifestations of cystic forms of spinal dysraphism depended on the localisation, size, anatomical variant, combination of anomalies, and type of complications encountered. The main clinical manifestations were motor disturbances (88.1%), pelvic dysfunction (76.7%), sensory disturbances (53.9%), trophic disturbances (39.7%), skin stigmata of dysembryogenesis (4.6%). However, to clarify the nature of the pathology of the spine, spinal cord, other organs and systems, and to understand polyvalent disorders, additional investigations were carried out.

Radiation methods are the most informative in the diagnosis of osteonephalic anomalies. The sensitivity and specificity of CT and MRI examinations in detecting spinal malformations is equal in the evaluation of bony and soft tissue masses, and the spinal cord. Computed tomography is a valuable method of imaging bony changes; MRI is the method of choice in the diagnosis of spinal malformations, associated intravertebral abnormalities and fixed spinal cord syndrome. When these techniques are used simultaneously, sensitivity and specificity reach 100%. Comprehensive studies showed that cystic forms of myelodysplasia were isolated in 140 (63.9%) observations; in 79(36.1%) they were combined with occult forms of spinal dysplasia. In the course of examination, various variants of osteoneural anomalies with involvement of the spine and spinal cord structures - neurospinal dysraphism and pathologies associated with changes in the spinal bone structures - lumbosacral dysraphism - were established. Myelodysplasias such as hydromyelia, diastematomyelia, syringomyelia, tetring - syndrome, lipomas, heterogeneous tissues were found in 53 (24.2%) patients at or cranial to herniated level. The frequency and variety of occult forms of myelodysplasia increased according to the severity of the anatomical variant and the degree of involvement of spinal cord structures. In 44(20%) cases, several combined anomalies were noted, aggravating the neurological consequences in the long term of treatment.

Motor disorders in 219 children with cystic spinal dysraphism were assessed using the five-point MRS (Modified Rankin Scale). The following scores were found in 88.1% of patients: 4 points in 9.3%; 3 points in 61.7%; 1- 2 points in 9.3%. In 19.7% of cases, no movement disorders were detected. Movement disorders were more intensely manifested in severe isolated forms of SMG in 94(48.7%) children; in combination of SMG with other spinal cord anomalies, in 79(40.9%); in spina bifida complicate, in 20(10.4%) patients. This can be explained by the fact that in severe and combined variants of osteonerval anomaly, the frequency of occult forms of spinal cord malformations tends to increase with increasing severity. In 45% of patients, motor disorders were accompanied by a number of other disorders: trophic changes in 34.5%; trophic disorders and joint deformities in 40.2%; joint deformities and trophic ulcers in 25.3%. The frequent combination of musculoskeletal, trophic disorders and deformities in the joints of the lower limb indicates common pathogenetic mechanisms.

In 57 (26%) patients with movement disorders, deforming arthrosis in the joints of the lower limbs, predominantly in the distal direction, was observed. Polymorphic paralytic foot deformities were detected in 47 (82.5%) patients. In 28 (59.6%) of them, they were bilateral with a predominant equinus component of the heel valgus or flat valgus deformity; in 19 (40.4%) they were unilateral. 3.6% of patients with severe osteoneural anomalies involving the thoracolumbar spine were bedridden. Out of 57(%) patients with various deformities, 24 (42.1%) had impaired movement due to subluxation or dislocation of the hip. 6 (10.53%) children had to move in a wheelchair due to absence or weakness of hip extensor and abductor muscles. 18 (31.58%) patients with severe peripheral paresis were able to stand with knee joints supported by the upper extremities. 33 (57.89%) children with various foot deformities walked with a limp on their own.

Such abnormalities occur because of a mismatch between the growth of the sheath and the spinal cord and spinal cord. This causes stretching of the nerve fibres, pinning them down by the strained dura mater. Disproportionate muscle traction, trophic effects, aggravating static-dynamic factors, aggravate deformities of the musculoskeletal system, lead to instability of vertical stability and movements in the lower extremities. Electromyography, performed in 128 patients, made it possible to establish the dependence of neuromuscular disorders on the level of damage of motor segments of the spinal cord.

Trophic disorders of lower limbs were revealed in 87 (45,1%) of 193 patients with cystic forms of spinal dysraphism who had motor disorders; in 45,1% of them vegetative-trophic disorders were revealed. In 20.7% of them chromata, shortening of the length and circumference of the lower extremities in the form of hypotrophy or atrophy of asymmetrical character were noted: on both sides - in 12 (66.7%) patients, on one side - in 6 (33.3%) patients. In 79.3% of children, a slight asymmetry of the lower limbs due to hypoplasia of the thigh or lower leg muscles was observed, which persisted as a residual condition in the long term after surgery. A severe consequence of trophic disorders is the formation of trophic ulcers. In 25.3% of patients with severe forms of spinal dysplasia or a combination of separate neurospinal and lumbosacral dysraphism, they resulted from the development of primary or secondary tethering syndrome. Trophic ulcers are chronically recurrent, increase in size, ooze deep-lying tissue, aggravate the course of the disease and reduce the potential for social maladjustment.

Pelvic organ dysfunction was noted in 270 (84.1%): spina bifida aperta in 168 and spina bifida occulta in 102. The nature and severity of urination and defecation disorders were assessed according to the established criteria and the results of special investigations. In 168 (52.3%) patients, the isolated or combined types of pelvic organ dysfunctions were caused by spinal malformations proper; in 102 (31.8%) they occurred in latent spinal dysraphism combined with anorectal, urogenital, and coloproctological anomalies. The severity and type of dysfunction depended on the nature of myelodysplasia, localization, and area of cleavage in the spine. In the main group 39(46,4%) children had hyperreflexive, 19(22,6%) - hyporeflexive, detrusor-sphincter dyssynergy - in 26(31%) types of the urinary dysfunction. Defecation disorder in the form of chronic constipation was observed in 27(42,8%) patients. Constipation combined with paradoxical faecal incontinence in 19 (30.2%) patients; anal sphincter insufficiency with faecal incontinence in 17 (27%) patients.

Isolated urinary disorders were observed in 84 (38.7%) patients; defecation disorders were observed in 63 (29%) in an isolated form. In 70 (32.3%) patients there was a combined defecation and urinary dysfunction.

Sensitivity disorders in cystic forms and latent spinal dysraphism were found in 131 (40.8%) patients with spina bifida aperta - in 118 (53.9%); with spina bifida occulta in association with malformations of other organs and systems - in 13 (12.7%). Pain sensitivity was investigated in 216 children under 3 years of age. From 3 to 7 years old - tactile and pain sensitivity (48 children). In 57 children 7 years and older superficial and deep sensitivity was assessed. Sensitivity disturbances were observed in both isolated and combined forms of myelodysplasia. They were pronounced in severe forms and were manifested by segmental, radicular changes in the form of hypoesthesia, and rarely by anaesthesia of the lower limbs and perineum.

Concealed spinal dysraphism is predominantly observed on the part of the spinal column in the form of vertebral anomalies, relatively rarely by spinal dysplasia or in various variants. Spina bifida occulta was detected in 102(31.8%) children. In isolated form without concomitant malformations - in 8 (7.84%); in association with anorectal - in 51(50%); urogenital - in 13 (12.75%); in 30(29.41%) patients - with colonic pathology accompanied by disorders of the act of defecation and urination. These abnormalities were presented in the form of flameless and fistulous forms of rectal atresia; cloaca, infravesical obstruction, renal and urinary tract malformations. Varieties of colonic pathology were congenital lengthening of the sigmoid colon - dolichosigma - in 7(23.3%); lengthening of the colon - dolichocolon - in 14(46.7%); lengthening and expansion of the whole colon - megadolichocolon - in 4(13.3%); expansion of the rectum - megarectum - in 5(16.7%). The presented data indicate that depending on the severity, nature and extent of latent spinal dysraphism, functional disturbances are observed in the zone of segmental innervation, often with abnormalities in the development of the corresponding organs and systems.

In SSD, cutaneous stigmata of dysembryogenesis were detected in 9.8% of cases. In anorectal and urogenital anomalies, cutaneous stigmata were observed frequently and varied according to malformations with more severe persistent functional disturbances than in patients with lengthening of various parts of the colon, accompanied by chronic colostasis.

Our observations indicate a high frequency of spinal pathology in the lumbosacral region. Functional and neurological disorders indicate the involvement of spinal structures in the area of their segmental innervation, which aggravates their course and negatively affects functional outcomes after surgery; therefore, targeted treatment of functional and residual disorders is necessary.

The type of SSD is verified by comprehensive functional and instrumental investigations. The main diagnostic methods for hidden spinal dysraphism are MRI and MSCT. Lumbosacral dysraphism (96.8%) in the form of postural abnormalities, non-invasion of the vertebral arches, anomalies of the bodies, sacrum, coccyx, or a combination of these anomalies predominated in the examined subjects. Rare (7.44%) spinal malformations such as spinal lipomas and tetring syndromes were also observed.

The nature of neurological disorders in SSD depends on the type and severity of the vertebral or spinal abnormalities, the form of the underlying abnormality for which the patient has received treatment. Different causal factors in the genesis of functional impairment cause differences in the intensity and nature of neurological disorders. This is confirmed by the presence of somatic, neurological and autonomic disorders in anorectal and urogenital anomalies and predominance of autonomic disorders with moderate or no somatic, neurological symptomatology in patients with colorectal anomalies.

The most unfavourable manifestation of SSD is pelvic disorders, which were detected in all 102 patients in the form of defecation, urination or a combination of both. In these patients, S I and SII segments of the spine responsible for the defecation and urinary functions were involved in the pathological process. The severity of the anorectal dysfunction depends on the nature and extent of the SSD, regardless of the form of ostensiviral dysfunction. In severe dysraphism, the dysfunction was more pronounced. However, the intensity and frequency of motor, sensory and orthopaedic dysfunction was less pronounced in SSD than in cystic spinal dysraphism.

Surgical treatment for cystic myelodysplasia is an indispensable part of comprehensive treatment. Of 219 patients, 198 (90.4%) underwent surgery. In 21 (9.6%) patients the pathology was considered incompatible with life. No surgical intervention was performed due to multiple anomalies. Surgical treatment in 20 (10.1%) patients was carried out at 1-28 days of age due to emergency indications. 103 (52.02%) patients were operated on routinely at the age of 1 month to 1 year, 69 (34.85%) at the age of 1-12 years. The surgery was greatly delayed in 6 (3.03%) patients aged 12-16 years. As our observations have shown, neurological manifestations progress after delayed surgery.

Osteonephalic anomalies are congenital. In an isolated form, they are rare; multiple lesions are more common, and the variant 'malformation due to malformation' is not excluded. In cystic forms of spinal dysraphism, malformations of other organs and systems were found in 32(14.6%); in SSD, in 14(13.7%). In single anorectal, urogenital, coloproctal anomalies or marked functional disturbances of these organs, the presence of other organs must be actively detected.

From 100 (31,2%) patients of comparison group, 6 patients had spinal dysraphism at the stage of follow-up; and 94 patients of the main group, after surgical intervention for correction of anorectal, urogenital and colorectal anomalies. Patients in this group required conservative, medical and physiotherapeutic treatment to correct functional abnormalities, with occult spinal pathology.

The analysis of our clinical material fully correlates with the recent literature on the feasibility of a comprehensive multidisciplinary approach to the diagnosis and verification of spinal malformations, including hidden forms, combined anomalies, and correction of secondary anthomo-functional disorders of other organs and systems.

The immediate and long-term results of treatment in terms of neurological status depend on the severity of myelodysplasia. Of the 77 (24%) patients in the comparison group, 68 (88.3%) patients had a dynamic neurological status of cystic forms. In 9 (11,6%) patients who were not included in the dynamic control group the pathology was considered inoperable, 3 (33,3%) of them died within 3-4 months after hospital discharge from various complications. No appreciable changes were found in 27 (51,9%) cases, in 17 (37,7%) a moderate positive dynamics of lower limb movements was revealed, in 8 (15,4%) cases negative dynamics was revealed. The treatment and diagnostic tactics corresponding to the functional disturbances were applied to the patients of the main group. The complex of treatment included preventive drug therapy (vascular, nootropic drugs, vitamin therapy) and physiotherapeutic procedures (massage, LFC, medicinal electrophoresis). Targeted treatment 2-3 weeks after surgery was given to patients with spinal malformations with the participation of a pediatric surgeon, urologist and orthopedist. In congenital spinal malformations, pelvic organ dysfunction is seen early in the child's life. Identification of the disorder and an individualised approach can improve the effectiveness of treatment. For bladder dysfunction, measures have been used to reduce the pressure in the hypertonic bladder or to increase the resistance of the bladder outlet to retain urine and increase bladder volume. In the hypotonic state, detrusor contractility was increased. In hyporeflexive detrusor dysfunction, continuous or periodic catheterization of the bladder at a certain time of the day was performed to decrease the bladder capacity, increase its sensitivity to distension and timely occurrence of urge to urination. To stimulate detrusor activity of the bladder, galantamine hydrobromide was prescribed (intramuscularly, in tablets, electrophoresis in the bladder area); sinusoidal modulated currents on the bladder area, physical therapy and general massage.

In the hyperreflexive type of urinary dysfunction, continuous catheterisation contributed to organ adaptation to an increase in the initial high intravesical pressure against a background of increased hydraulic pressure. Physiological solution with antibiotics or furacilin 1:5000 solution in an amount of 50% of the organ's age capacity was injected into the bladder through the catheter. The catheter was closed for four hours, then the bladder was emptied completely and the total contents measured. The difference between injected and excreted fluid was used to determine the bladder capacity and the volume of the child's diuresis in four hours. During 7-10 days in the first half of the day (from 8 to 24 hours) the manipulation was repeated every 4 hours, increasing the injected liquid by 10 ml. In the second half of the day (from 24 to 8 a.m.) the catheter was closed. The course of treatment was repeated after three months. Complex drug therapy included m-cholinolytics, atropine by electrophoresis in the bladder area for 5 days, driptan 2.5-5 mg 2-3 times daily for 1-2 months, sedative therapy at bedtime (novopassit, motherwort) in an age-dependent dose. Drug therapy was combined with physiotherapy, electrophoresis with m-cholinolytics, electrotherapy and low-energy laser.

In detrusor-sphincter dyssynergia, medication and physiotherapy treatment was the same as for the hyperreflexive type.

For defecation disorders in the form of constipation, special importance was given to regular emptying of the rectum at certain times of the day. A dietary therapy was chosen in an induvidical manner. Olive, linseed and sunflower oils were used. Stimulation with galantamine - hydrobromide was given intramuscularly during 10 days, further on - in the form of tablets during 30-40 days. To strengthen the abdominal press and perineum muscles, therapeutic gymnastics, tonic massage of the anterior abdominal wall, long back and lumbar muscles and laser therapy were performed; dysbacteriosis correction was prescribed. In defecation disorders with anal sphincter insufficiency phenomena therapeutic measures aimed at training and strengthening of rectal retention apparatus were used: purging and training enemas with gradual increase of fluid infusion and prolongation of retention time in rectum; electrical stimulation of sphincter apparatus and mechanical training on a rubber tube.

When defecation disorders are combined with urinary disorders, the treatment was aimed at correcting the defecation disorder.

Motor disorders, symmetrical or asymmetrical deformities and pathologies of the lower limb joints, trophic disorders, instability of vertical stability and movement occur due to imbalance of muscle traction and force imbalance between the muscular antagonist and synergist groups due to spinal innervation disorders. These abnormalities are less pronounced in most young patients. Against the background of comprehensive basic therapy, repeated courses of massage, physiotherapeutic procedures and staged plaster correction provide better results with less residual phenomena.

The effectiveness of the multidisciplinary approach is confirmed by the positive results of the treatment of patients with occult spinal dysraphism combined with abnormalities of other organs and systems, and the reduction of functional disorders of the relevant organs.

Among patients in the comparison group and in the main group, neurological disorders were either unchanged or had a positive or negative shift during the treatment phases. Trophic disorders tended to progress, sensitive ones were more stable. With systematic courses of supportive therapy, patients in the main group showed positive dynamics in the motor sphere and in pelvic organ dysfunction. This fact confirms the expediency of the outpatient observation of patients, repeated 10-15 day courses of treatment in an outpatient clinic or hospital every 3-4 months for 2 years, and later - 2 times a year.

The effectiveness of the proposed diagnostic and therapeutic tactics has been confirmed by comparative analyses of survival rates and treatment outcomes in both groups.

CONCLUSIONS

1. Vertebromedullary anomalies in children, localized in 68% of cases in the lumbosacral spine, manifest in different anatomical forms either isolated (63.9%) or in combination (36.1%); differ morphologically and structurally in the form of cystic cleavage involving the membrane and substance of the spinal cord - myelodysplasia (68.2%) and latent spinal dysraphism with predominant bone-component disorders (31.8%) combined with abnormalities of other organs and systems with overt or obliterated neurological manifestations.

2. The spectrum and severity of the clinical and neurological manifestations of spinal dysraphism depend on the level of neurosegmental damage, the extent and the nature of myelodysplasia. The course is worsened by the association of vertebromedullary anomalies and the occurrence of secondary complications.

3. The polymorphism and nonspecificity of the clinical manifestations of spinal dysraphism are due to the presence of hidden forms of myelodysplasia and vertebral abnormalities, a high frequency of malformations of other organs and systems, mutually aggravating the course and quality of life of patients. This necessitates a comprehensive diagnostic approach to their detection.

4. In vertebromedullary anomalies the leading clinical syndromes are pelvic organ dysfunction (84.1%), motor (73.8%), sensory (40.8%), autonomic (19.3%) and trophic disorders (39.7%), cutaneous disembryogenesis (6.2%), rarely cranial nerve damage and signs of mental retardation (22.4%).

5. Latent forms of spinal dysplasia occur as additional malformations of the spinal cord in anatomical variants of spina bifida aperta, sometimes transforming into spinal cord fixation syndrome or invisible vertebromedullary anomalies with neurological and functional impairments; abnormal shape and structure of the organs concerned (anorectal and urogenital system) in the area of their segmental innervation.

6. The genesis of progressive neurological and residual disorders after surgery for spinal malformations is dominated by "fixed spinal cord" syndrome, which

was present before surgery as a combined congenital pathology or due to an adhesive process associated with surgery.

7. The severity and type of pelvic organ dysfunction depend on the nature of the myelodysplasia and the localisation and area of cleavage in the spine. The main manifestations are constipation (42.8%), faecal incontinence (27%), constipation combined with paradoxical incontinence (30.2%) and urinary disorders (hyperreflexive (46.4%), hyporeflexive (22.6%), detrusor-sphincter dysfunction (31%))alone or in combination.

8. Inadequate diagnostic and therapeutic tactics in some specialist hospitals (neurosurgical, surgical, neurological) for spinal pathology fail to identify the nature of concomitant pathology and secondary changes of a functional and organic nature in other organs, improve treatment outcomes and improve patients' quality of life.

9. Optimisation of diagnosis to identify the nature of spinal pathology, active detection and early targeted treatment of secondary disorders associated with spinal dysraphism, with the involvement of appropriate specialists, has improved the immediate and long-term results of treatment of patients in the core group.

PRACTICAL GUIDANCE

The early diagnosis of CSD depends above all on the alertness of paediatricians and doctors in other specialties to this pathology. The detection of skin stigmata in the lumbosacral region, progression of neurological symptoms, pelvic organ dysfunction, orthopaedic disorders, anorectal, urogenital and colorectal abnormalities are indications for the diagnosis of occult spinal dysraphism.

Comprehensive diagnosis of vertebromedullary anomalies reveals subclinical neurological abnormalities and structural and functional conditions of the organs involved. Radiological methods are the main diagnostic methods. CT and MRI studies have a sensitivity and specificity of up to 100%.

A spinal MSCT combined with an excretory urography or contrast-enhanced irrigography can assess the spine, the urinary tract and the colon at the same time.

Urogenital and coloproctal anomalies should be considered as markers of co-morbid osteonephalous anomalies.

Surgical treatment of children with spinal malformations should be carried out in specialised institutions. Postoperatively, children with spinal malformations should be monitored by allied specialists and undergo repeated courses of rehabilitation therapy.

REFERENCE LIST

1. Abdullaeva M. E. Features of physical development and thermoregulation of children in the first year of life (longitudinal study): Autoref. diss. Candidate of medical sciences. - T., 2003. - 22 c.

2. Abishev B. H., Mukhametzhanova S. V., Meiramova A.K., Osintsev K.A. Modern methods of radial diagnosis of spinal development anomalies // VII Polenovsky readings: Proc. Saint-Petersburg, 2008. - C. 314.

3. Averianov A. I. Glazkova I. V. Krasnov A. V. Alekhine K. V. A case of early prenatal diagnosis of diastematomyelia // Prenat. Diagnostic. - 2008. - Vol. 1, No.4. - C. 73-76

4. Alyaev Y. G. G., Grigoryan V. A., Gadzhieva Z. K. Urinary disorders. - Moscow: Litterra, 2006. - 208 c.

5. Al Absi Esmat Abdulrashid Mahmoud Radial diagnosis of malformations of the caudal spinal cord and spine in childhood: Author's dissertation. D. in medical sciences. - Saint Petersburg, 2009. - 22 c.

6. Antonova I. V., Bogacheva E. V., Filippov G. P., Lyubavina A. E. The role of exogenous factors in the formation of congenital malformations of the fetus // Voprosy of gynecology, obstetrics and perinatology. - 2010. - Vol. 9, №6. - C. 63-68.

7. Antonov O. V., Katina M.M., Artyukova S.I., Gorbacheva E. M. Epidemiological study of congenital malformations of the nervous system // Polenovsky readings: Proc. of All-Russian scientific and practical conference - Saint Petersburg, 2010. - C. 304.

8. Akhmediev M. M., Vakkasov N. Y., Akhmediev T. M. Treatment of neurogenic pain syndromes due to fixed spinal cord // Neurology. - Tashkent, 2013. - №2. - C. 103-104.

9. Akhmediev M. M., Yugay I. A., Vakkasov N. Y., Ahmediev T. M. Classification and diagnosis of hydrocephalus in children with congenital spinal hernias // Journal of Theoretical and Clinical Medicine. - Tashkent,

2014. - N5J120145. - C. 54-58.

10. Akhmediev M. M. Neuroprotection in the correction of neurological disorders in children with spinal hernias : a scientific publication / M. M. Akhmediev // Neurology. - Tashkent, 2012. - N3-4. - C. 205

11. Akhmediev M. M. Surgical treatment and quality of life in children with congenital spinal hernias: a scientific publication / M. M. Akhmediev, N. Y. Vakkasov, T. M. Akhmediev // Journal of Theoretical and Clinical Medicine. - Tashkent, 2013. - N4 J120134. - C. 112-116.

12. Akhmediev M.M., Makhmudov Sh.D. Diagnosis of abnormal development of the spine and spinal cord in newborns and children in the first year of life // Neurosurgery and Neurology of Kazakhstan. - Almaty, 2009. - №2-3. - C. 55-56.

13. Akhmediev M.M., Makhmudov Sh.D., Shamsiev A.T. Congenital spinal hernias in children and their surgical treatment // International Journal of Neurology. - Moscow, 2009. - Vol. 30, № 8. - C. 53-56.

14. Akhmediev M.M., Makhmudov Sh.D. Radiology and diagnostic criteria for surgical treatment of children with spinal hernias // III Eurasian Radiology Forum "Radiology: Science and Practice": Proceedings. - Astana, 2009. - C. 413-415.

15. Akhmediev M.M., Makhmudov Sh.D. The course and prognosis of surgical treatment of congenital spinal hernias in children // Polenevsky readings: Proc. All-Russian Scientific and Practical Conf. 22-24 April 2009. - Saint-Petersburg, 2009. - C. 317.

16. Akhmediev M.M., Mahmudov Sh.D., Vakkasov N.Y., Akhmedieva Sh.R. Historical perspective in the treatment of congenital spinal hernia with concomitant hydrocephalus // Materials of the IV Scientific-Practical Conference with international participation "Actual problems of neurosurgery". - Tashkent, 2010. - C. 21-23.

17. Akhmediev M.M., Mahmudov Sh.D., Vakkasov N.Y., Akhmedieva Sh.R. Complex treatment of congenital malformations of the primary neu-

ral tube in children // Proceedings of the Scientific and Practical Conference of Neurosurgeons of Ukraine with the participation of the Scientific Research Institute of Neurosurgery named after acad. Burdenko N.N. "Problems of Reconstructive and Reconstructive Neurosurgery. - Autonomous Republic of Crimea, 2010. - C. 11.

18. Akhmedieva Sh.R., Akhmediev M.M. Fixed-brain syndrome in children with spinal dysraphia // Achievements, problems and prospects of child and adolescent health care: Proceedings of the Republican Scientific and Practical Conference. 25 March 2010. - Tashkent, 2010. - C. 27-29.

19. Baindurashvili A. G. Ivanov S. V. Kenis V. M. Hip subluxation and dislocation in children with consequences of spinal hernia (literature review) // J. Traumatology and Orthopaedics of Russia. - 2013. - Vol. 70, No. 4. - C. 97-102.

20. Bekheladze I.D. Esetov M.A. Diastematomyelia: possibilities of three-dimensional echography // Prenatal Diagnostics. - 2009. - Vol. 8, no. 2. - C. 45-47.

21. Bogdanov E. I. Bladder dysfunction in organic diseases of the nervous system // Bekhterev Neurological Bulletin. V. M. Bekhterev. - 2009. - C. 2-10.

22. Buriev M.N. Umurtka pogonasining tugma nuksonlarini aniklashda multislite computer tomographada tekshirishning ahamiyati // Materials of the scientific-practical conference "Actual problems of neurosurgery". - Tashkent, 2008. - C. 18.

23. Burkhanov V.V. Osipov I.B., Lebedev D.A. Results of surgical treatment of urinary incontinence in children with neurogenic bladder dysfunction // Bulletin of St. Petersburg University. - 2008. №11. - C. 187-194.

24. Vakkasov N.Y. Dynamics of neurological deficit in the postoperative period with congenital spinal hernia Proceedings of the IV Scientific-Practical Conference with International Participation "Actual problems of neurosurgery". Tashkent, 2010. - C. 23-24.

25. Vakkasov N.Y., Khodiev A.A., Madaminjanov U.O. The role of neurosonography in the diagnosis and treatment of congenital spinal hernias // Proceedings of the IV Scientific-Practical Conference with international participation "Actual problems of neurosurgery". - Tashkent, 2010. - C. 201-202.

26. Vakkasov N.Y., Akhmediev M.M., Akhmedieva Sh.R. Causal factors in the development of spinal hernia in children. Materials of the Republican Scientific-Practical Conference "Medical and Organizational Aspects of Care for Children and Adolescents". - Tashkent, 2011. - C. 147-148.

27. Vissarionov S. V., Golubev K. E., Belyanchikov S. M. Complex treatment of a patient with multiple malformations of the spine and spinal cord // Traumatology and Orthopaedics. - 2011. - Vol. 62, No 4. - C. 95-99.

28. Vishnevsky E.L. Neurogenic bladder dysfunction. In the book Pediatric surgery: a national guide / edited by: Y.F. Isakov, A.F. Dronov. Moscow: GEOTAR-Media, 2009. - C. 634-643.

29. Voronov V. G., Syrchin E. F., Zyabrov A. A., Ivanov A. A., Potemkina E. G., Pershin V. A. Fixed spinal cord syndrome: current views on etiology and pathogenesis, clinical presentation, diagnosis and treatment (review of scientific publications) // Scientific and practical journal "Neurology and neurosurgery of childhood. - 2011. - №2. - C. 53-61.

30. Voronov V.G., Chmutin E. G. Vertebromedullary malformations in childhood: A practical guide to the diagnosis and treatment of malformations of the spinal cord and spine in childhood // - M.: Econ-Inform Publishing House, 2016. - 395 c.

31. Guk M.Y., Stashkevich A.T., Orlov Y.O. Neuroorthopaedic manifestations of spinal hernias depending on the form and level of the lesion // Bulletin of Orthopaedics, Traumatology and Prosthetics. - 2008. - №1. - C. 17-22.

32. Gaiduk Y. V. Clinical polymorphism of neurological symptoms in

congenital malformations of the spine and dysplastic scoliosis in children: Author's dissertation. D. in medical sciences. - Saint Petersburg, 2009. - 24 c.

33. Gaiduk Y. V., Sharina I. E. Features of nervous system disorders in congenital lesions of the musculoskeletal system and malformations of the spinal cord. // Scientific and Practical Journal "Clinical and Laboratory Consilium. - 2010. - C. 123-125.

34. Grigoryeva E.V. Possibilities of radiodiagnostics in the assessment of surgical interventions in children with spinal cord and spinal cord developmental anomalies: Author's dissertation. D. in medical sciences. - Moscow, 2004. - 24 c.

35. Gulyamova M.K., Shamsurov Sh., Mutailoeva D.S. Risk factors in the development of spinal pathology in young children. VI Congress of Pediatricians of Uzbekistan. - 2009. - 56 c.

36. Damulin I. V. The use of Niwalin In neurological practice. - 2009. - C. 1 - 7.

37. Demyanenko V.A., Kabanyan A.B., Baydakov A.P., Ermakov S.V., Firsov A.L. Diagnosis, treatment tactics of types of occult dysraphism (spina bifida occulta): dorsal dermal sinus, fixed spinal cord // Kubanskiy scientific medical herald. - 2012. - №6. - C. 85-87.

38. Diyarov N.A. The course and results of surgical treatment of spinal hernias in neonates and infants: Author's dissertation. Diyarov N.A., Doctor of medical sciences. - Tashkent, 2007. - 22 c.

39. Degtyareva E.I., Baindurashvili A.G., Konyukhov M.P. Types of locomotor dysfunction in children with paralytic foot deformities in the aftermath of spinal lumbosacral hernias // Traumatology and Orthopaedics of Russia. - 2009. - №2(52). - C. 81-87.

40. The epidemiology and early diagnosis of congenital malformations of the spine and spinal cord // Voprosy sovremennoi pediatrii. - 2008. - №4. - C. 58-61.

41. Elikbaev G.M. Congenital spinal hernias in children // Polenov Readings Materials of the All-Russian Scientific-Practical Conference dedicated to the 150th anniversary of V.M. Bekhterev. - Saint Petersburg, 2007. - C. 263-264.

42. Elikbaev G.M. Complex approach to methods of examination of children with myelodysplasia // Polenov Readings Theses of the All-Russian Scientific and Practical Conference. - Saint-Petersburg, 2009. - C. 324.

43. Elikbaev G.M., Khachatryan V.A. Karabekov A.K. Congenital spinal pathologies in children. - Shymkent, 2008. - C. 80.

44. Efremenko A.D., Nikolaev S.N. Treatment of trophic osteomyelitis in children with malformations of the caudal spine and spinal cord // J. Traumatology and Orthopaedics Russia. - 2009. - №2(52) - 2009. - C. 85-89.

45. Zyabrov A.A., Syrchin E.F., Bain B.N., Ivanov A.A.. Voronov V.G. Diagnostic significance of ENMG in patients with spinal dysraphism // Polenov readings Theses of the All-Russian scientific and practical conference. - Saint-Petersburg, 2009. - C. 324.

46. Zyabrov A.A., Voronov V.G., Ivanov A.A., Syrchin E.F. To the question of neurogenic bladder variants in CNS malformations // Polenov Readings All-Russian Scientific and Practical Conference: Proc. -St. Petersburg, 2009. - C. 325.

47. Zyabrov A.A., Syrchin E.F., Voronov V.G., Kutumov E.B., Al-Absi E. Clinic, diagnosis of "Fixed spinal cord syndrome" in caudal spinal dysraphia in childhood // Polenov Readings Theses of All-Russian Scientific and Practical Conference - Saint Petersburg, 2009. - C. 325-326.

48. Zyabrov A.A., Voronov V.G., Syrchin E.F., Ivanov A.A., Kutumov E.B. Pershin V.A. Clinic and treatment of spina bifida occulta // Polenov Readings Materials of the All-Russian Scientific and Practical Conference. - Saint Petersburg, 2010. - C.311-312.

49. Zykov V. P., Akhmadov T.Z., Nesterova S.I., Safonov V. A Diagno-

sis and treatment of motor disorders in young children EF // Pediatrics, 2011. - Special issue of Diseases of the nervous system. - C. 32-35.

50. Ignatiev R.O., 2003; Khachatryan V.A., Orlov Y.A., Osipov I.B., Elikbaev G. M. Spinal dysraphia: Neurosurgical and neuro-urological aspects. - SPb: Dyatka, 2009. - 304 c.

51. Ivanov S. V., Kenis V. M. Radiological features of the hip joint in children with consequences of spinal hernia // Genius of Orthopaedics - 2011. - №1. - C. 93-97.

52. Ilyin A. V., Syrchin E. F., Bain B. N. Cost-effectiveness analysis in children operated on for spinal hernia // VII Polenov Readings Theses of the All-Russian Scientific and Practical Conference. -St. Petersburg, 2008. - C. 327 - 328.

53. Ismoilov Z.N., Mirjuraev E.M., Tilavov S.U. Pyramid yulining pathologiyasi bulgan bolalarning tibbiy rehabilitacida nivalin dori vositassining kullashning samaradorligi. "Bolalar va usmirlarga tibbiy yordam cadetishning tibbiy-tashkili kirralari", Respublika ilmiy-amali anjumani materialari, Toshkent, 2011, P.172 -173.

54. Kadyrbekov N.R. Surgical correction in the treatment of children with spina bifida in conditions of insufficient epithelialization of the hernia sac shell : scientific publication / N.R. Kadyrbekov, I.A. Yugay // Achievements and prospects of specialized medical care for children (Uzbek model): collection of abstracts of international conference (2015, Tashkent). - Tashkent, 2015. - C. 47

55. Kariev G.M., Akhmediev M.M., Akhmedieva Sh.R. Developmental anomalies of the spine and spinal cord in early life // Darmon. - February 2010. - № 2 (53). - C. 6-9.

56. Kolesnikova N.G. Anorectal dysfunction in lumbosacral vertebral arch failure: Avoref. diss. ... Candidate of Medical Sciences. - Saint Petersburg. 2004, - C. 24.

57. Kubrina M.V., Melnik T.N., Tarasova O.V. A case of ultrasound diagnosis of terminal myelocystocele in a newborn // Journal of Prenatal Diagnostics. - 2016. - Vol. 15, No. 2. - C. 175-178.

58. Kuznetsova T.V. Etiopathogenetic and clinical features of the course of cerebrospinal hernias in children, improvement of methods of surgical correction and rehabilitation. Author's abstract of the dissertation. Candidate of medical sciences. D. in medical sciences. - Bishkek, 2008. - 24 c.

59. Kushel Y.V., Zemlyansky M.Y. Syndrome of 'secondary fixation of the spinal cord' after correction of various forms of spinal dysraphism in children // Neurosurgery. - 2010. - № 2. - C. 41-46.

60. Lazishvili M.N. Efferent methods of treatment of neurogenic urinary dysfunction in children with myelodysplasia syndrome: Author's dissertation. D. in medical sciences. - Moscow, 2014.

61. Larkin I.I. Acute and chronic vertebro-medullary insufficiency in spinal injuries, tumours and deformities in children : Author's dissertation. D. in medical sciences. - Omsk, 2009.

62. Mamayunusov Sh. Sh., Urinov Sh. U. Features of Diagnosis and Surgical Treatment of Congenital Spinal Hernias // Materials of the Scientific and Practical Conference "Actual Problems of Neurosurgery". - Tashkent, 2008. - C 28-29.

63. Martynenko A.A. Surgical treatment of children with spinal hernias (prenatal and postnatal diagnosis and surgical correction): Author's abstract. D. in medical sciences. - Perm, 2010. - C. 24.

64. Martynenko A.A., Pisklakov A.V., Bardeeva K.A., Krupko N.L. Surgical treatment tactics of children with spinal hernias depending on the cleavage rate // Russian bulletin of pediatric surgery, anesthesiology and intensive care. - 2011. - №2, - C.133-137.

65. Matveeva SP, Semenov PN, Lutsik AA Clinical and diagnostic characteristics of congenital malformations of the spinal cord and spine // Polenev Readings Materials of the All-Russian Scientific and Practical

Conference dedicated to the 150th anniversary of V.M. Bekhterov. - Saint-Petersburg, 2007. - C. 273.

66. Matchanova A.T. The role of perinatal diagnosis of congenital malformations in reducing perinatal losses: Author's abstract. Candidate of medical sciences. - T., 2004 - 26 p.

67. Makhmudov Sh.D., Akhmediev M.M., Yugay I.A. Ultrasonography in the diagnosis of spinal hernias combined with hydrocephalus // Achievements, problems and prospects of child and adolescent health care. The results of the Republican Scientific-Practical Conference on 25 March 2010. - Tashkent, 2010. - C. 49-51.

68. Makhmudov Sh.D., Akhmediev M.M., Yugay I.A. Reconstructive surgery in children with congenital spinal hernias // Proceedings of the IV Scientific-Practical Conference with international participation "Actual problems of neurosurgery". - Tashkent, 2010. - C. 32.

69. Makhmudov Sh.D., Akhmediev M.M., Yugay I.A., Pak S.I. Modern radiological diagnosis of spinal dysraphia // VIII scientific-practical conference of radiologists of Uzbekistan "Modern methods of medical imaging and interventional radiology", 22-23 April 2010. - Coll. of papers. - Tashkent. - C. 173-174.

70. Mendelevich E. G. Syringomyelia: a comprehensive clinical MR tomographic and MRI morphometric study: Author's dissertation. D. in medical sciences. - Kazan, 2002. - C. 26.

71. Mirzayan E.I. Disability due to congenital anomalies in children in the Russian Federation and peculiarities of medical and social rehabilitation: Ph. Candidate of medical sciences. - Moscow, 2011. - C. 3-20.

72. Nikitin S.V. Diastematomyelia as a concomitant threshold of the spine // Prenatal Diagnostics. - 2008. - Vol. 7, No. 4.

73. Nikolaev S.G. Workshop on clinical electromyography : textbook. - Saint Petersburg, 2004. - C. 45 -63.

74. Nikolaev S.N. Spinal bladder: In the book Pediatric Surgery: a national manual. - Moscow: GEOTAR-Media, - 2009. - C. 625-634.

75. Ovsova O.V. Clinical and epidemiological analysis and risk factor assessment of congenital malformations of the central nervous system in children: Author's dissertation. D. in medical sciences. - Ekaterinburg, 2007. - C. 5-24.

76. Orlov Y.A., Protsenko I.P., Marushchenko L.L. Adaptation capabilities of children operated on in infancy for hydrocephalus // Polenov Readings Materials of the All-Russian Scientific and Practical Conference. - Saint-Petersburg, 2010. - C. 330-331.

77. Orlov Y.A., Plavsky P.N., Plavsky N.V. Spinal hernias complicated by liquorrhea // Polenov Readings. Materials of All-Russian Scientific and Practical Conference. - Saint-Petersburg, 2010. - C. 330- 337

78. Osipov I.B., Khachatryan V.A., Sarychev S.A., Elikbaev G.M. Diagnosis and treatment of myelodysplasia in children with urological complications // Pediatrics and Pediatric Surgery of Kazakhstan. - 2008, - №1. - C. 14-17.

79. Pavlov A.Y., Romikh V.V., Moskaleva N.G. Urinary bladder dysfunction in children: some issues of diagnosis and ways of effective therapy // Pediatrics, - 2007. - Vol. 86, No. 5, - P. 51-54.

80. Pak A.I., Larkin I.I., Larkin V.I., Preobrazhensky A.S. Value of ENMG in determining the severity of spinal cord injury in children // V Congress of Russian Neurosurgeons, - Ufa, 2009, - P. 329.

81. Pankova Ye.E., Matulevich S.A., Golikhina T.A., Klipa M.V. Monitoring of congenital malformations in the system of evaluation of prenatal diagnosis in Krasnodar region // Kuban Medical Journal. - 2010. - C. 150 - 154.

82. Pisklakov A.V. Combined pelvic organ dysfunctions in children (principles of prenatal and postnatal functional and neurophysiological diagnosis and surgical treatment: Author's dissertation. D. medical sciences.-

Omsk, 2007. - C. 28.

83. Potolova E. V. Application of modern ultrasound technology for early diagnosis of fetal spinal hernia: a scientific publication // Ultrasound and Functional Diagnostics. - M., 2013. - №4. - C. 120

84. Prityko A.G. Possibilities of surgical treatment of urinary incontinence in children with congenital malformations of the spine and spinal cord / A.G. Prityko, I.V. Burkov, S.N. Nikolaev et al. // Pediatric Surgery. - 1997. - № 1. - C. 47 - 51.

85. Pugachev A.G., Pugacheva V.I. Urinary incontinence. In Children's Urology: A Guide for Physicians. - Moscow: GEOTAR-Media, - 2009. - C. 521-531.

86. Pullman N.F. Clinical and pathogenetic characteristics of infectious diseases of the spinal cord in children: Ph. - Moscow, 2004. - C. 3 - 28.

87. Reimbayev A.Y., Aliev M.A., Makhmudov Sh.D. Radiation diagnosis methods in congenital spinal hernias // Proceedings of the IV Scientific-Practical Conference with international participation "Actual problems of neurosurgery". - Tashkent, 2010. - C. 208-209.

88. Rizaeva N.T. Shamansurov Sh., Nurmatova D.A. Features of the clinical course of enuresis in patients with neurogenic bladder // Proceedings of the VI Congress of Pediatricians of the Republic of Uzbekistan. - 2009. - C. 202.

89. Rudakova A.V., Larionov S.N. Features of diagnosis and treatment of spinal malformations in childhood // Bulletin of the All-Russian Scientific Center of the Russian Academy of Medical Sciences, - 2012. - Vol. 86, no. 4. - Part 2. - C. 122-125.

90. Rudakova A.V., Larionov S.N., Sorokovikov V.A. "Fixed" spinal cord (Literature review) // Bulletin of All-Russian Scientific Center of RAMS. - 2011. - Vol. 80, 4. - Part 1. - C. 348 - 353.

91. Rudakova A.V., Larionov S.N., Sorokovikov V.A. Gruzin P.G., Byankin V.F. Some features of diagnosis and treatment of osteoneural

dysplasia - "Fixed spinal cord" // Bulletin of All-Russian Scientific Center of the Russian Academy of Medical Sciences. - 2010. - Vol. 75, №5. - C. 119-120.

92. Savin D.M. Surgical treatment of patients with spinal deformities against the background of spinal dysraphia. D. thesis. D. in medical sciences. - Kurgan, 2016. - C. 145.

93. Sebelev K.I., Al-Absi E.A.M., Voronov V.G. Diagnosis and surgical treatment of children with enuresis in spina bifida occulta // Polenevsky readings. Materials of All-Russian Scientific-Practical Conference dedicated to the 150th anniversary since the birth of V.M. Bekhterov, - St. Petersburg, 2007, - p. 284 -285.

94. Soprunova I. V., Belopasov V. V., Tkacheva N. V. Spinal hernia prevalence in the Astrakhan region, outcomes and prevention // Medical Herald of the North Caucasus, - 2012. - №1. - C. 72-74.

95. Syrchin E.F., Bain B.N., Voronov V.G. Development of a quality of life assessment scale for children operated on for spinal hernia // Medical Almanac. - 2012. - Vol. 24, No. 5. - C. 112 - 116.

96. Syrchin E.F., Zyabrov A.A., Voronov V.G., Kutumov E.B., Ivanov A.A., Pershin V.A. Associated myelomeningocele with hydromyelia and syringomyelia // Polenovsky readings Materials of the All-Russian Scientific and Practical Conference, - Saint Petersburg, 2010. - C. 339-340.

97. Syrchin E.F. Fixed spinal cord syndrome in caudal spine and spinal cord dysraphia in children: Author's dissertation. D. in Philosophy. - Perm, 2005. - C. 28.

98. Sysoev K. V. Prognosis of surgical treatment of fixed spinal cord syndrome in children: Ph. D. in medical sciences. - Saint Petersburg, 2017. - C. 28.

99. Sysoev K.V. Zharova E.N., Zabrodskaya Y.M. et al. Latent fixed spinal cord syndrome in children (clinical observation and review of the literature) // Neurosurgery. - 2016. - №2. - C. 53-58.

100.Sysoev K.V., Semenova J.B., Larionov S.N. et al. // Pediatric neurosurgery: clinical guidelines / edited by S.K. Gorelishev - Moscow. 2016. - C. 266-283.

101. Sysoev K.V., Nazinkina Y.V., Khachatryan V.A. 3-Tl MR tractography of caudal spinal cords in various forms of spinal dysraphia in children // Radiation Diagnostics and Therapy. - 2016. - №2 - C. 52 - 57.

102.Trifonova K. P. Physical rehabilitation of children with concomitant spinal cord and spinal cord injury: Author's dissertation. D. in medical sciences. - Moscow, 2009. - 26 c.

103. Ulrikh E.V. , Voronin D.V. , Guseva I. A. , Kemkin V. B. , Kolesnikova N. G., Krutelev N.A., M.A. Mushkin , , S.A. Sarychev . [5], Sarychev S.A. , Snischuk V. P. , Yalfimov A. N. // Split spinal cord syndrome (diastematomyelia): A training manual. - St. Petersburg, 2012. - 196 c.

104.   Ulrich, E.V. Vertebrology in terms, figures, pictures / E.V. Ulrich, A.Yu. Mushkin. - SPb. ELBI-SPb, 2004. - 187 c.

105. Usmonkhonov O. A., Mirsadykov D.A., Makhmudov M. M. Features of surgical treatment of spinal hernias in children // Materials of the Scientific and Practical Conference "Actual problems of neurosurgery". - Tashkent, 2008. - C. 49 - 50.

106. Khachatryan V.A., Elikbaev G.M. Myelodysplasia in children: features of diagnosis and clinic // Journal of neurosurgery and neurology of Kazakhstan -2009 - [1],-P. 15-23.

107. Khachatryan V.A., Orlov Y.A., Osipov I.B. Spinal dysraphia: neurosurgical and neuro-urological aspects // St. Petersburg: Dyatka, 2009. - 304 c.

108. Khodykin, E.A. Excitability threshold of spinal cord roots during electrostimulation as an additional criterion for the prognosis of surgical treatment of spinal cord anomalies in children / E.A. Khodykin, K.V. Sysoev, V.A. Khachatrian // Bulletin of Clinical Neurophysiology. - 2016.

- №1 (4). - С. 71 - 75.

109.   Khachatryan V.A., Sysoev K.V. On topical problems of pathogenesis, diagnosis and treatment of fixed spinal cord syndrome (analytical review) // Neurosurgery and Neurology of Childhood. - 2014. - №3. - С. 76 - 87.

110.   Shamsiev A.M., Atakulov D.O., Aliev B.P., Mutalibov I.A., Zainiev S.S. Diagnosis and surgical treatment of spinal hernias in newborns // U11 Polenov Readings Theses of the All-Russian Scientific and Practical Conference. - Saint Petersburg, 2008. - С..356.

111.   Shapkova E. Yu. // Rehabilitation of children with spinal cord injuries: A training manual. - Moscow, 2004. - 185 с.

112.   Shodiev A.Sh., Mamadaliev A.M., Choriev U.H., Nabiev A.A. On the feasibility of using a new surgical method in the treatment of spinal hernias // Materials of scientific and practical conference "Actual problems of neurosurgery". - Tashkent, 2008. - С. 56.

113.   Shodiev A.Sh., Aliev M.A., Ravshanov N.D. Frequency and medical and social consequences of congenital neurosurgical malformations // Polenov Readings Theses of the All-Russian Scientific and Practical Conference. - Saint-Petersburg, 2009. - С. 355.

114.   Shamansurov Sh. Shamansurov, M.K. Gulyamova, D.S. Mutailoeva // Neurology. - Tashkent, 2010. - №1. - С. 7-11

115.   Shomansurov Sh., Ohunboeva D.A., Rizaeva N.T. Clinical, neurological and computed tomographic parameters in patients with znuresis on the background of minimal spinal insufficiency // Neurology, - 2005, - № 4, - P. 2-3.

116.   Shchepin O.P., Korotkikh R.V., Tregubov Y.G. Prevention in the XXI Century: Analysis of Conceptual Approaches // Problems of Social Hygiene, Public Health and History of Medicine. - 2009. - №4. - С. 3-7.

117.   Yugay I. A. A. Craniospinal pressure correction in the treatment of hydrocephalus combined with spinal hernias: a scientific publication / I.A.

Yugay, M.M. Akhmediev, Sh.D. Mahmudov // Achievements, problems and prospects of child and adolescent health: Proceedings of the Republican Scientific and Practical Conference (Tashkent, March 25, 2010). - Tashkent, 2010. - C. 163-164

118. Yugay I.A., Akhmediev M.M. Management of children with hydrocephalus combined with spinal hernias // Polenov Readings Theses of the All-Russian Scientific and Practical Conference. - Saint Petersburg, 2009, - P. 355 - 356.

119.   Yugay I.A., Akhmediev M.M., Mahmudov Sh.D., Tulaev N.B. Opportunities of magnetic resonance imaging in spinal dysraphic diseases // VIII scientific-practical conference of radiologists of Uzbekistan "Modern methods of medical imaging and interventional radiology", 22-23 April 2010. - Coll. of papers. - Tashkent. - C. 322-323.

120. Yugay I.A., Akhmediev M.M., Makhmudov Sh.D. Craniospinal pressure correction in treatment of hydrocephalus combined with spinal hernias // Polenov Readings Materials of the All-Russian Scientific and Practical Conference. - Saint Petersburg, 2010, - P. 345.

121. Ergashev N.Sh., Diyarov N.A. Justification of complex treatment tactics for spinal hernias in newborns. // Materials of the Scientific and Practical Conference "Actual problems of neurosurgery". Tashkent, 2008, P 58 - 59.

122.   Ergashev N.Sh., Diyarov N.A. Ismanalieva M.M. Therapeutic tactics for spinal hernias in neonates with open hydrocephalus syndrome // Materials of the Scientific and Practical Conference "Topical problems of neurosurgery". - Tashkent, 2008. - C. 57 - 58.

123. Ergashev N.Sh. Otamurodov F.A. Ergasheva N.N. Nurmatov D.S. Tastanov A.M. Anomalies of the spine and spinal cord in children with anorectal malformations // Journal of Theoretical and Clinical Medicine. - 2018. - №1. - C. 75-79.

124. Eshonkhojaeva K.O., Osmanov R.Y., Atalikov A.I. Some issues of

diagnosis and treatment of congenital spinal hernias in children // Bulletin of the Association of Doctors of Uzbekistan. - 2007. - №2, - C. 50-52.

125. Adzick N.S, Thom E.A, Spong C.Y, et al. A randomized trial of prenatal versus postnatal repair of myelomeningocele // N Engl J Med. - 2011. - Vol. 364. - P. 993-1004.

126. Adzick N.S. Fetal myelomeningocele: natural history, pathophysiology, and in-utero intervention // Semin Fetal Neonatal Med. - 2010. - Vol. 15. - P. 9-14.

127. Agata Korzeniecka Kozerska, Bożena Okurowska Zawada, Joanna Michaluk Skutnik, Anna Wasilewska. The Assessment of Thiol Status in Children with Neurogenic Bladder Caused by Meningomyelocele // Urology Journal - 2014. Vol. 11, № 02. - P.1400-1404.

128. Aldana P.R, Wood D.L, Postlethwait R.A, James H.E. Initiating, developing and evaluating a comprehensive spinal defects clinic: a clinical report. Pediatr Neurosurg. - 2010. - Vol. 46, №5. - P. 329-334.

129. Alexander G McNeil, Sandhya Jose, Chris Rowland-Hill // Diastematomyelia in a 3-year-old girl. Images in paediatrics (August 28, 2017). http://dx.doi.org/10.1136/archdischild-2017-313281.

130. Ali MZ. Cystic spinal dysraphism of the cervical region: experience with eight cases including double cervical and lumbosacral meningoceles // Pediatr Neurosurg. - 2010. - Vol. 46, №1. - P. 29-33.

131. Ann Flanagan, Marianne Gorzkowski, Haluk Altiok, Sahar Hassani, Kwang Woo Ahn. Activity Level, Functional Health, and Quality of Life of Children with Myelomeningocele as Perceived by Parents // Clin Orthop Relat Res. - 2011. - Vol. 469. - P. 1230-1235

132. Anthony P. Trenga, Anuj Singla, Mark A. Feger, Mark F. Abel Patterns of congenital bony spinal deformity and associated neural anomalies on X-ray and magnetic resonance imaging. Journal of Children's Orthopaedics. Published Online:1 Aug. - 2016 https://doi.org/10.1007/s11832-016-0752-6.

133. Bademci G., Saygun M. Batay F.et al. Prevalence of primarytethered cord syndrome associated with occult spinal dysraphism in primary school children in Turkey // Pediatr. Neurosurg. - 2006. - Vol.42, no. 1. - P. 13-17.

134. Blondiaux E, Katorza E, Rosenblatt J, Nahama-Allouche C, Lenoir M, le Pointe HD, Garel C. Prenatal US evaluation of the spinal cord using high-frequency linear transducers // Pediatr Radiol. - 2011. - Vol. 41, №3. - P. 374-383.

135. Börcek A.Ö, Ocal O, Emmez H Split cord malformation: experience from a tertiary referral centre // Pediatr Neurosurg. - 2012. - Vol. 48. - P. 291-298.

136. Boulet S.L, Yang Q, Mai C, Kirby R.S, Collins J.S, Robbins J.M, et al. Trends in the postfortification prevalence of spina bifda and anencephaly in the United States // Birth Defects Res A Clin Mol Teratol. - 2008. - Vol. 82. - P. 527-532.

137. Byung-Jou Lee, Moon-Jun Sohn, Seong-Rok Han, Chan-Young Choi, Dong-Joon Lee, Jae Heon Kang. Analysis of Risk Factors and Management of Cerebrospinal Fluid Morbidity in the Treatment of Spinal Dysraphism // J Korean Neurosurg Soc. 54. - 2013. - P. 225-231.

138. Cheng B., Li, F. T. Lin L. SPINE Diastematomyelia // Journalof Bone and Joint Surgery, doi:10.1302/0301-620X.94B3. 2012;94-B:365-72.

139. Chong Hyeok Yoon, Sang Kyu Kang, Chan Hee Jin, Moon Sun Park, Jeong Hoon Rho A meningomyelocele with normal intracranial signs on ultrasound and false-negative amniotic fuid alpha-fetoprotein and acetylcholinesterase // Obstet Gynecol Sci. - 2014. - Vol. 57, №3. - P. 223-227.

140. Chong Hyeok Yoon, Sang Kyu Kang, Chan Hee Jin, Moon Sun Park, Jeong Hoon Rho // A meningomyelocele with normal intracranial signs on ultrasound and false-negative amniotic fuid alpha-fetoprotein and

acetylcholinesterase Obstet Gynecol Sci. 2014. - Vol. 57, №3. - P. 223-227.

141. Cools M.J, Al-Holou W.N, Stetler W.R Jr, Wilson T.J, Muraszko K.M, Ibrahim M, et al. Filum terminale lipomas: imaging prevalence, natural history, and conus position / J Neurosurg Pediatr. - 2014. - Vol. 13, №5. - P. 559-567.

142. Cornips E.M, Vereijken I.M, Beuls E.A, Weber J.W, Soudant D.L, van Rhijn L.W, et al. Clinical characteristics and surgical outcome in 25 cases of childhood tight filum syndrome // Eur J Paediatr Neurol. - 2012. - Vol. 16, №2. - P. 103-117.

143. Czeizel Andrew E, Zolta´n Ba´rtfai and Ferenc Ba´nhidy. Primary prevention of neural-tube defects and some other congenital abnormalities by folic acid and multivitamins: history, missed opportunities and challenges. // The Author(s), 2011. Reprints and permissions: http: //www.sagepub.co.uk/journals Permissions.nav.P. 173 - 188.

144. Danzer E, Gerdes M, Bebbington MW, et al. Lower extremity neuromotor function and short-term ambulatory potential following in utero myelomeningocele surgery // Fetal Diagn Ther. - 2009. - Vol. 25. - P. 47-53.

145. Danzer E, Johnson M.P, Bebbington M, et al. Fetal head biometry assessed by fetal magnetic resonance imaging following in utero myelomeningocele repair // Fetal Diagn Ther. - 2007. - Vol. 22, №1-6. [PubMed: 17003546].

146. Dhaulakhandi D.B, Rohilla S, Rattan K.N. Neural tube defects: review ofexperimental evidence on stem cell therapy and newer treatment options // Fetal Diagn Ther. - 2010. - Vol. 28, №2. - P. 72-78.

147. Di Cesare A., Leva E, Maccini F.et al. Anorectal malformations and neurocpinal dysraphism: is this association a major risk for continence? // Pediatr.Surg, Int. - 2010. - Vol. 26. - P.1077-1081.

148. Dorothea Stiefel, Andrew J. Copp, and Martin Meuli. Fetal spina bi-

fida: Loss of neural function in utero // J Neurosurg. Author manuscript; available in PMC 2013. - P. 1-12.

149.   Drew Alexander Bednar, Cauda equina syndrome from lumbar disc herniation // CMAJ. - 2016. - Vol. 188, no. 4: 10.1503/cmaj.150206 PMCID: PMC4771539 PMID: 26504103

150. Erhan Arslan, Kayhan Kuzeyli, Elif Acar Arslan. Intraspinal lipomas without associated spinal dysraphism // Iran Red Crescent Med J. - 2014. - Vol. 16, №5. - P 1- 4.

151.   Fariborz Samini, Hosein Mashhadinejad, Mahdi Khajavi, Mohammad Samini // Orthopaedic Lesions in Tethered Cord Syndrome: The Importance of Early Diagnosis and Treatment on Patient Outcome. Arch Bone Joint Surg. - 2014. - Vol. 2, №2. - P. 93-97. http://abjs.mums.ac.ir the online version of this article abjs.mums.ac.ir

152. Georg Thieme Verlag KG Stuttgart Screening and Treatment of Tethered Spinal Cord in Anorectal Malformation Patients // Eur J Pediatr Surg New York. - 2016. - Vol. 26, no. 01. 022-028DOI: 10.1055/s-0035-1563673

153. Gerhauser I, Geburek F, Wohlsein P. Perosomus elumbis, cerebral aplasia, and spina bifida in an aborted Thoroughbred foal // Res Vet Sci. - 2010 Dec 10.

154. Glenn C, Cheema A.A, Safavi-Abbasi S, et al. Spinal cord detethering in children with tethered cord syndrome and Chiari type 1 malformations // J Clin Neurosci. - 2015. - Vol. 22. - P. 1749-1752.

155. Gluncic V, Turner M, Burrowes D, et al. Concurrent Chiari decompression and spinal cord untethering in children: feasibility in a small case series // Acta Neurochir (Wien). - 2011. - Vol. 153. - P. 109-114. Discussion 114.

156. Graciela Manucci, Enzo von Quednow. How I Do It: Neural Tube Defects in Guatemala - Myelomeningocele Spina Bifida Unit Como Lo Hago Yo: Anomalías del Tubo Neural en Guatemala - Mielomeningocele

Unidad de Espina Bífida e Hidrocefalia // SNI: Pediatric Neurosurgery. - 2014. - Vol 5. - P. 13-22.

157. Hauger O, Obeid I, Pelé E. [Imaging of the fused spine] // J Radiol. - 2010. - Vol. 91. - P. 1035-48.

158. Hosny I.A, Elghawabi H.S. Ultrafast MRI of the fetus: an increasingly important tool in prenatal diagnosis of congenital anomalies. Magn Reson Imaging. - 2010. - Vol. 28, №10. - 1431-1439.

159. Hsien-Yi Chiu, Yi-Hua Liao. Occult Spinal Dysraphism // The New England Journal of Medicine. September. - 2014. - P. 465-466.

160. Jamie D Olesen, Darcie A Kiddoo, Peter D Metcalfe The association between urinary continence and quality of life in paediatric patients with spina bifida and tethered cord // Paediatr Child Health. - 2013. - Vol.18, no.7. - P. 32-35.

161. José Murillo B. Netto, André N. Bastos, André A. Figueiredo, Luis M. Pérez, Spinal Dysraphism: A Neurosurgical Review for the Urologist. - 2009. - Vol. 11, № 2. - P.71-79.

162. Kang J.K., Yoon K.J., Ha S.S. et al. Surgical management and outcome of tethered cord syndrome in school aged children, adolescents, and young adults // J. Korean. Neurosurg. Soc. - 2009. - Vol. 46. - P. 468-471.

163. Katherine Ottolinia, Amy B. Harrisb, June K. Amlingb, Ann M. Kennellyb, Leslie A. Phillipsb Laura L. Tosia. Wound care challenges in children and adults with spina bifida: An open-cohort study // Journal of Pediatric Rehabilitation Medicine: An Interdisciplinary Approach 6. - 2013. - P.1-10 .

164. Khan Y. A, Batool T, Rasool N, Jahan Y, Habib Q, Saddal N. S. Anterior sacral meningocele // J Coll Physicians Surg Pak. - 2010. - Vol. 20, №5. - P. 337-338.

165. Kıymaz N, Yılmaz N, Güdü BO, Demir I, Kozan A. Cervical spinal dysraphism. Pediatr Neurosurg. - 2010. - Vol. 46, №5. - P. 351-356

166. Kondo A, Kamihira O, Ozawa H. Neural tube de fects: prevalence,

etiology and prevention // Int J Urol. - 2009. - Vol. 16. - P. 49-57.

167. Krista S, Owen Devine, Ling Hao, Nicole F, Song Li, Anne M Molloy, Zhu Li, Jianghui Zhu, Robert J Berry. Population red blood cell folate concentrations for prevention of neural tube defects: a bayesian model // BMJ. - 2014. - Vol. 349. - P.1-12.

168. Kural C, Guresci S, Simsek G.G, Arslan E, Tehli O, Solmaz I, et al. Histological structure of filum terminale in human fetuses // J Neurosurg Pediatr. 2014. - Vol. 13, №4. - P. 362-367.

169. KushelIuV, Zemlianskiĭ M. Iu, Khit' M. A. Tethered cord syndrome in different types of spina bifida in children // Zh Vopr Neirokhir Im N N Burdenko. - 2010. - Vol. 2. - P. 19-23.

170. Lan Z.G., Richard S.A., Lei C, Huang S. Thoracolumbar spinal neurenteric cyst with tethered cord syndrome and extreme cervical lordosis in a child: A case report and literature review // Medicine (Baltimore). - 2018. - Vol. 97, №16. e 0489. doi: 10.1097/MD.0010489. PMID: 29668630.

171. Liu L, Li J, Huang S, You C. Adult anterior sacral meningoceles misdiagnosed as pelvic cysts // Br J Neurosurg. - 2011 Feb 23.

172. Liu W, Zheng D, Cui S, et al. Characteristics of osseous septum of split cord malformation in patients presenting with scoliosis: a retrospective study of 48 cases // Pediatr Neurosurg. - 2009. - Vol. 45. - P. 350-353.

173. Lora Kahn, MD, Nnenna Mbabuike, MD, Edison P. Valle-Giler, MD,Juanita Garces Fetal Surgery: The Ochsner Experience with In Utero Spina Bifida Repair // The Ochsner Journal. - 2014. - P. 112-117.

174. Maiti T.K, Bhat D.I, Devi B.I, Sampath S, Mahadevan A, Shankar S.K. Teratoma in split cord malformation: an unusual association: a report of two cases with a review of the literature // Pediatr Neurosurg. - 2010. - Vol. 46, №3. - P. 238-241.

175. Milhorat T.H, Bolognese P.A, Nishikawa M, et al. Association of Chiari malformation type I and tethered cord syndrome: preliminary re-

sults of sectioning filum terminale // Surg Neurol. - 2009. - P. 20-35.

176. Mohammad Jafar Golalipour, Mostafa Qorbani, Arezo Mirfazeli, Elham Mobasheri. Risk factors of neural tube defects in Northern Iran // Iran Red Crescent Med J. - 2014. - Vol. 16, №6. - P. 1-5.

177. Mooney J.F. Concurrent orthopaedic and neurosurgical procedures in pediatric patients with spinal deformity / J.F. Mooney, S.S. Glazier, W.R. Barfield // J Pediatr Orthop. - 2012. - Vol. 21 (6). - P. 602-605.

178. Morimoto K., Takemoto O., Wakayama A. Spinal lipomas in children-surgical management and long-term follow-up // Pediatr. Neurosurg. - 2005. - Vol. 41. - P. 84-87).

179. Mukesh Shukla, Jayesh Sardhara, Rabi Narayan Sahu, Pradeep Sharma, Sanjay Behari, Awadesh Kumar Jaiswal, Arun Kumar Srivastava Adult versus pediatric tethered cord syndrome: Clinicoradiological differences and its management // Asian journal of neurosurgery. Year: - 2018, Vol. 13, Issue: 2, - P. 264-270.

180. Muller-Godeffroy E., MichaelT,Poster M, Seidel U, Schwarke D, Thyen U. Self-reported health-related quality of life in children and adolescents with myelomeningocele // Dev Med Child Neurol. - 2008. - Vol. - P. 456-461.

181. Mustafa Barutcuoglu, Mehmet Selcuki, Ahmet Sukru Umur, Mesut Mete, Seren Gulsen Gurgen, Deniz Selcuki. Scoliosis may be the first symptom of the tethered spinal cord // Indian journal of orthopaedics Year: - 2016, Issue: 1. - P. 80-86

182. Nikhil Nair, M Sreenivas, Arun K Gupta, Devasenathipathy Kandasamy, Manisha Jana Neonatal and infantile spinal sonography: A useful investigation often underutilized // Pediatric. New Delhi, India, Year: - 2016. Vol. 26, Issue: 4, - P. 493-501.

183. Oucheng N, Lauwers F, Gollogly J, Draper L, Joly B, Roux FE. Frontoethmoidal meningoencephalocele: appraisal of 200 operated cases // J Neurosurg Pediatr. - 2010. - Vol. 6, №6. - P. 541-549.

184. Rao Z.X, Li J, Hang S.Q, You C. Congenital spinal intradural arachnoid cyst associated with intrathoracic meningocele in a child. J Zhejiang Univ Sci B. - 2010. - Vol. 11, №6. - P. 429-432.

185. Romagna, A. Detethering of a congenital tethered cord in adult patients: an outcome analysis / A. Romagna, B. Suchorska, C. Schwartz et al. // Acta neurochir (Wien). - 2013. - Vol. 155 (5) - P. 793-800.

186. Scott N. Adzick Fetal myelomeningocele: natural history, pathophysiology, and in-utero intervention // Semin Fetal Neonatal Med. - 2010. - Vol. 15, №1. - P. 9-14.

187. Scott N., Adzick, M.D., Elizabeth A. Thom, Ph.D., Catherine Y. Spong, M.D., John W. Brock III, M.D., Pamela K. Burrows, M.S., Mark P. Johnson, M.D., Lori J. Howell, R.N., M.S., Jody A. Farrell, R.N., M.S.N., Mary E. Dabrowiak. A Randomized Trial of Prenatal versus Postnatal Repair of Myelomeningocele // N Engl J Med. Author manuscript; available in PMC. - 2013. - Vol. 11. - P. 1-15.

188. Sean Barry Quality of Life and Myelomeningocele: An Ethical and Evidence-Based analysis of the groningen protocol // Pediatr Neurosurg. - 2010. - Vol. 46. - P. 409-414.

189. Sepulveda W, Wong A.E, Sepulveda S, Corral E. Fetal Scalp Cyst or Small Meningocele: Differential Diagnosis with Three-Dimensional Ultrasound // Fetal Diagn Ther. - 2011 Jan 6. [Epub ahead of print] PubMed PMID: 21212653.

190. Seyed Ali Alamdaran, Najmeh Mohammadpanah, Samira Zabihian, Mohammad Esmaeeli Diagnostic value of ultrasonography in spinal abnormalities among children with neurogenic bladder // Electron Physician. - 2017. - Vol. 9, №6. - P. 4571-4576.

191. Stanescu Ioana, Kallo Rita, Bulboaca Adriana, Dogaru Gabriela. Role of rehabilitation a case of diastematomyelia // Balneo Research Journal DOI: http://dx.doi.org/10.12680/balneo. - 2017. - Vol. 8, №4, P. 227 - 230

192. Sudhansu Sekhar Mishra, Souvagya Panigrahi, Manmath Kumar Dhir, and Deepak Kumar Parida Tethered cord syndrome in adolescents: Report of two cases and review of literature // J Pediatr Neurosci. - 2013. - Vol. 8, №1. - P. 55-58.

193. Sumi A, Sato Y, Kakui K, Tatsumi K, Fujiwara H, Konishi I. Prenatal diagnosis of anterior sacral meningocele // Ultrasound Obstet Gynecol. - 2011. - Vol. 37, №4. - P. 493-496.

194. Talamonti G., D'Aliberti G., Collice M. Myelomeningocele: long - term neurosurgical treatment and follow - up in 202 pa tients // J. Neurosurg. Neurosurg. Pediatrics. - 2008. - Vol. 107, № 5. - Suppl. - P. 368- 386.

195. Tereza Cristina Carbonari de Faria, Sergio Cavalheiro.// Improvement of motor function and decreased need for postnatal shunting in children who have undergone intrauterine myelomeningocele repair // Arq Neuropsiquiatr. - 2013. - Vol. 71(9-A). - P. 604-608).

196. Theofanakis C, Theodora M, Sindos M, Daskalakis G. Prenatal diagnosis of sirenomelia with anencephaly and craniorachischisis totalis: A case report study. Copyright © 2017 The Authors. Published by Wolters Kluwer Health, Inc. All rights reserved.PMID: 29390297 PMCID: PMC5815709

197. Tu A, Steinbok P. Occult tethered cord syndrome: a review // Childs Nerv Syst. - 2013. - Vol. 29, №9. - P. 1635-1640.

198. Tulipan N, Sutton LN, Bruner J. P, Cohen B.M, Johnson M, Adzick NS. The effect of intrauterine myelomeningocele repair on the incidence of shunt-dependent hydrocephalus // Pediatr Neurosurg. - 2003. - Vol. 38. - P. 27-33.

199. Tungaria A, Srivastav A.K, Mahapatra A.K, Kumar R. Multiple neural tube defects in the same patient with no neurological deficit // J Pediatr Neurosci. - 2010. - Vol. 5, №1. - P. 52-54.

200. Uddanapalli Sreeramulu Srinivasan, Natarajan Raghunathan, Law-

rence Radhi Long Term Outcome of Non-Dysrhoaphic Intramedullary Spinal Cord Lipomas in Adults // Case Series and Review Asian Spine J. - 2014. - Vol. 8, №4. - P. 476-483

201. Vidmer S, Sergio C, Veronica S, et al. The neurophysiological balance in Chiari type 1 malformation (CM1), tethered cord and related syndromes // Neurol Sci. - 2011. - Vol. 32. - P. 311-316.

202. Wykes, V. Asymptomatic lumbosacral lipomas--a natural history study / V. 120 Wykes, D. Desai, D.N. Thompson // Childs Nerv Syst. - 2012. - Vol. 28 (10). - P. 1731-1739.

203. Yelikbayev G. M. Tutayeva A. A. Clinical Manifestation of A Tethered Cord Syndrome in Children. M, Tutayeva A. A. Clinical Manifestation of A Tethered Cord Syndrome at Children and Research Methods for Early Diagnosis of Disease. Biomed Pharmacol J 2015;8(2): http://biomedpharmajournal.org/p=3850

204. Yong R.L. Symptomatic retethering of the spinal cord following section of a tight filum terminale / R.L. Yong, T.H. Habrock-Bach, Vaughan M. et al. // Neurosurgery. - 2011. - Vol. 68. - P. 1594-1602.

205. ZdzisA'aw Kawecki, Alicja Fara, StanisÅ'aw Kwiatkowski, Laura Mary Åczak, Olga Milczarek, Tomasz Kwiatkowski, Izabela Herman-Sucharska. Tethered cord syndrome in children. Journal of Orthopaedics Trauma Surgery and Related Research.2017. - Vol. 49. - P.67.

206. Zhou, Yuan M.D; Zhu, Lin M.D; Lin, Yixing M.D; Cheng, Huilin M.D, Chiari type I malformation with occult tethered cord syndrome in a child // A case report. Medicine: - 2017. - Vol. 96. - Issue 40. - P 8239.

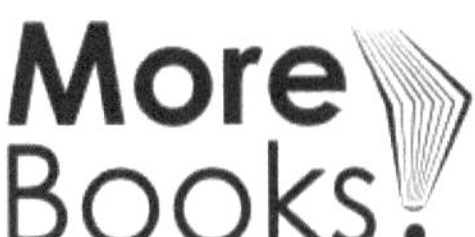

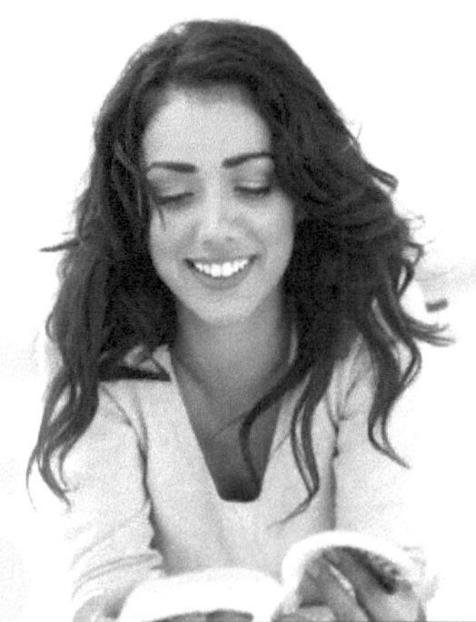

I **want** morebooks!

Buy your books fast and straightforward online - at one of world's fastest growing online book stores! Environmentally sound due to Print-on-Demand technologies.

Buy your books online at
www.morebooks.shop

Kaufen Sie Ihre Bücher schnell und unkompliziert online – auf einer der am schnellsten wachsenden Buchhandelsplattformen weltweit! Dank Print-On-Demand umwelt- und ressourcenschonend produzi ert.

Bücher schneller online kaufen
www.morebooks.shop

KS OmniScriptum Publishing
Brivibas gatve 197
LV-1039 Riga, Latvia
Telefax: +371 686 204 55

info@omniscriptum.com
www.omniscriptum.com

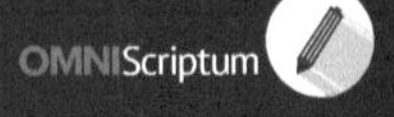

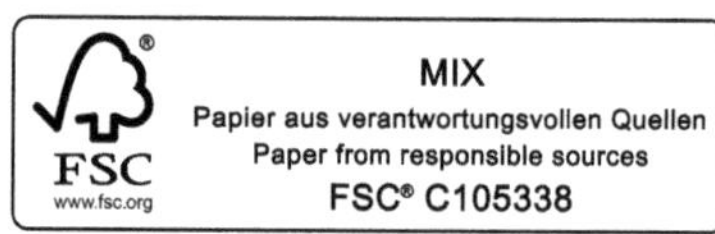

Printed by Books on Demand GmbH, Norderstedt / Germany